Dinesh Palipana OAM is a doctor, lawyer, disability advocate, and researcher. He has a spinal cord injury with quadriplegia affecting the use of his fingers, parts of the arms, and everything below the chest.

He became the first medical graduate with quadriplegia in Queensland, then the first graduate doctor with quadriplegia to begin work in the state. He was the second graduating doctor with quadriplegia to start working clinically in Australia.

Dinesh obtained a medical degree from Griffith University and a law degree from Queensland University of Technology. He has completed an advanced clerkship in radiology at Harvard University where to their knowledge, he was the first visiting student with quadriplegia.

Dinesh was the 2021 Queensland Australian of the Year. He was awarded an Order of Australia Medal in 2019 and was the third Australian to receive a Henry Viscardi Achievement Award in New York, awarded in 2019.

Dinesh was born in Sri Lanka, then moved to Australia at the age of 10. He resides in Gold Coast, Australia. Dinesh works at the Gold Coast University Hospital and Griffith University. He is close to his mother, Chithrani. He enjoys motorcars, anything with an engine, music – mostly hip-hop from the 90s and 2000s – chocolate and adventure.

Dinesh Palipana
STRONGER

MACMILLAN
Pan Macmillan Australia

Pan Macmillan acknowledges the Traditional Custodians of country throughout Australia and their connections to lands, waters and communities. We pay our respect to Elders past and present and extend that respect to all Aboriginal and Torres Strait Islander peoples today. We honour more than sixty thousand years of storytelling, art and culture.

Some of the people in this book have had their names changed to protect their identities.

First published 2022 in Macmillan Australia by Pan Macmillan Australia Pty Ltd
1 Market Street, Sydney, New South Wales, Australia, 2000

 A catalogue record for this book is available from the National Library of Australia

Typeset in 12.5/18 pt Adobe Garamond Pro by Post Pre-press Group, Brisbane

Printed by IVE

The author and the publisher have made every effort to contact copyright holders for material used in this book. Any person or organisation that may have been overlooked should contact the publisher.

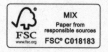 The paper in this book is FSC® certified. FSC® promotes environmentally responsible, socially beneficial and economically viable management of the world's forests.

This book is dedicated to my mother,
Chithrani Palipana.

Mum, you have made me who I am today.
Thank you for your unconditional courage, sacrifice,
patience, strength and love.

CONTENTS

INTRODUCTION

OVER THE YEARS, a lot of friends have talked to me about writing this book: the story of my life and the things I've learned as I've lived it. Still, I always wondered whether it would be arrogant of me to think that anyone would want to read my story. One of my closest friends eventually said, 'I never read books, but I would read one about your life.' Coming from a man who never reads, this made me think that maybe there was something to the idea. Maybe there was something worth sharing about this journey.

My journey has been first and foremost that just of a human being. I think that this is important, because I've learned that labels don't matter. Our titles don't matter. They are artificial. Transient. Vulnerable to the whims of society. Social status can be fleeting. Worldly belongings aren't forever. All can be lost in seconds, and I know this too well. What matters is our humanity – what we do and who we are when all these things are taken away. That's what can connect us most to the universe, ourselves, and our fellow humans. And, truth be told, we are connected in a way that transcends all of our differences. The butterfly effect. Six degrees of separation. Well, 6.6 according to some studies.

But if I had to use some labels, I would say that today I'm a doctor in an emergency department. It's Australia's busiest emergency department, in fact. I've qualified as a lawyer, become a researcher in spinal cord injury and am proudly a disability advocate. I've been told that I am most likely the first person in Australia, maybe even the world, to do this combination of things with my characteristics. I am a son to an awesome mother – the best, in my opinion. I am the boyfriend of an amazing woman, one who is intelligent, beautiful and caring. I like music, mostly old rap. I like cars or, well, anything with an engine. I like to do things like paramotoring, jet boating, skydiving and anything else that might raise the heart rate. I like chocolate. I have a spinal cord injury with quadriplegia. It's probably this last bit that really makes my journey a little bit different from others.

Notwithstanding that, my journey still hasn't been linear. I was born in Sri Lanka. The country had a gross domestic product (GDP, which is the amount of finished goods and services made within a country) of about US$6 billion at the time. Although contentious, the GDP is sometimes touted as a measure of living standards and economic progress. At the age of 10, I moved to Australia, a country with nearly the same population as Sri Lanka but a GDP about 32 times greater. In geographical terms, Australia is 117 times bigger. Sri Lanka experienced a prolonged period of civil war, while Australians have had peace on home soil for a long time. Moving between the two countries was like moving between two different worlds.

I've lived through depression, a spinal cord injury, and a series of things that have made life a roller-coaster ride. Has life been hard? No. I don't see it that way, mostly because I know that there are many in this world who have had a harder life. I'm not the kid in Africa who walks miles to have a sip of water, not knowing what the world will bring them tomorrow. I'm not the person with a disability stuck in a war zone, unable to escape the bombs, hoping that death will not come. I'm not the one who never had an opportunity to learn to read. No, I'm still the lucky one.

I'm grateful for the journey I've had so far. It's made me who I am. Even though I might not have always seen it at the time, the hard times have been ultimately good for me. After all, you can't make a sword without forging metal in a fire.

In telling you about my travels through these different experiences, there are just four main thoughts that I want to share with you. First, no matter how hard things get, it's going to be okay. It has been for me. It will be for you.

Second, life doesn't have to be linear. Even if you want it to be, it's probably not going to be. As Robert Burns said, the best laid schemes of mice and men often go awry.

Third, a linear life is boring anyway. Isn't a squiggle more interesting than a straight line? Think of all the movies about ships. They are full of adventure. Would you prefer a story about the ship making an uneventful journey from one port to another, or one that must weather storms and even a mutiny? Come to think of it, I can't recall any celebrated story about an uneventful journey from one port to another.

Finally, as you experience all this, know that you are more resilient than you think. Believe that. Don't bow down. Make your life your life.

Here we are then. I'm writing the stories which will hopefully convince you that these ideas hold true. Let's take a look through my life, where the me of today will tell you about the things I learned from the me of yesterday. If you're not convinced, that's okay – at least my friend who doesn't read will have read a book.

Where do I start, though? Do I go through the obligatory early years? It feels like a boring thing to do – for me, if not for you. I considered skipping ahead to more interesting parts. But another one of my closest friends said, 'No, you need to lay down the foundation first.'

I suppose that the present makes a whole lot more sense when you understand the past. So, here it is. I'll start from the very beginning.

1

THE BEGINNING
OF THE BEGINNING

Whatever happens to you has been waiting to happen
since the beginning of time.

Marcus Aurelius

WE ONCE DID a genetic test on my family. It's amazing how
much a little bit of saliva can tell you. We sent a sample in
a kit to the company by mail. After a few weeks, the results
turned up on their website. The test showed the likelihood
of the owner of the DNA having certain conditions; for
example, it said I was at increased risk of coeliac disease.
This was true, because I do indeed have the condition as
confirmed by the normal tests. I actually feel fortunate
to have coeliac disease. I've eaten far less junk food since
I was diagnosed. If it wasn't for coeliac disease, I might
be writing this book to you as the heaviest doctor on
earth. Still, I thank the lord they make gluten-free pizza.

The DNA test also checked whether I'm a carrier for diseases like cystic fibrosis, which I'm not. There were some other interesting results too, like whether or not I'm a deep sleeper. Although these findings may not be backed by solid science yet, it correctly identified that I'm not a deep sleeper.

I think we sometimes fail to appreciate how rapidly technology moves. Over a period of about 15 years, DNA sequencing went from costing over $100 million to less than $1000 per human genome, and now takes a fraction of the original processing time. $100 million. That's a lot of pizza. My entire genome was sequenced for $99 over a matter of days somewhere around 2014. That's over 3 billion pairs of letters that makes me who I am, on a computer somewhere. Maybe someone will use the data to clone people one day – even another me.

The test also traced our family history. My mum has genes from all over the world. There was even some American Indian heritage in her ancestry. I have no idea how such a cosmopolitan mix of blood made it into a small town in Sri Lanka. We must've had some frisky ancestors who roamed the planet. Dad's ancestry was concentrated in South India and Sri Lanka. When these two lineages converged, the result was me. I popped out in 1984. I was the treasured and only child of Chithrani and Sanath Palipana. I was born on the same day as Christopher Reeve. Superman. Until much later, I had no idea how similar our journeys would be.

My mum, Chithrani, has shaped my life in uncountable ways. I'll tell you more about her as we go. But what you should know up front is that she has made me who I am. No matter what idea I had, she always said that it was possible. No dream was too big, no vision too bold. She has always believed in me. She has made so many sacrifices for me, including eventually her marriage to my dad. Even when everyone walked away, this woman has always been there with me. She's five foot two inches in height, but giant in will.

When I was growing up, Sri Lanka was experiencing a difficult period in its history. The civil war between the Sinhalese and Tamil people raged from 1983 to 2009. It's said that the war had its origins in Sri Lanka's colonial English past, which led to a series of events that caused the conflict. That aside, what's important is that between 80,000 and 100,000 people are estimated to have died. Inside that war, there was also a communist uprising between 1987 and 1989. The insurrection was started by a Marxist movement led by a guy who at one point went to medical school in Russia, a story very similar to Che Guevara. The group was aptly nicknamed the 'Che Guevara Clique' by Sri Lankan intelligence agencies. Although he didn't finish studying to become a doctor, he affected the history of an entire nation. This insurrection resulted in the death of tens of thousands more people.

Isn't it curious how we can read those numbers so objectively? Even perhaps with a level of detachment.

100,000 people.

That's 100,000 dreams; 100,000 daily routines; 100,000 memories of a lifetime. 100,000 people with families. 100,000 people who were loved by someone – a brother, a mother, a grandparent. It's even more thought-provoking that these numbers sometimes don't even make the headlines. They're simply a side note, giving precedence to the messy divorce of a socialite who's famous for the sake of being famous.

I have a striking memory from those days. I was sitting on Mum's lap in the front seat of a grey four-wheel drive. Yes, it was world-class road safety in the rural Sri Lanka of the eighties. We were driving along a winding road in a remote area. In the distance, I saw thin columns of black smoke rising like serpents into the sky. The atmosphere felt sinister. I could almost smell the danger. The air was thick with it. As we got closer, the source of the smoke became visible. There were tall stacks of tyres lining the sides of the road, on fire. Inside those tyres were people. They were being burned alive.

For so many years, I knew this memory but never thought much about it. In my 30s, I started to question it. You know those memories that your mind sometimes embellishes? Was it that? I wondered, was it even real? Was it just something I saw on TV? I finally asked my mum about it, and she said that the horrific vision of that day really happened. She went on to ask, 'Do you remember what you saw next?' I didn't. What was next were the heads of people on stakes lining the road, after they were beheaded.

This was life for many people back then. Parents were afraid to go to work on the same bus in case it was blown up. They deliberately took separate buses, so at least one of them made it home for the kids. I lost an uncle who fought in the war. I watched his wife and little son cry at the funeral. A young war widow with her child who was too young to understand the world that he lived in. It was the first time that death became a real and palpable concept to me.

Some have told me not to talk about the trouble Sri Lanka once had. They feel that it paints the country in a bad light. I don't agree. I think it's important to understand the history of a nation, because this informs the future it can build. The world has had holocausts, pogroms and apartheid. We've learned and grown after them, or at least tried to. Without acknowledgement of the mistakes made and the lessons learned, nations cannot move forward and thrive. After a while, Sri Lanka became a far cry from the nation it was during the time of the civil war. Around the mid-2010s, it was even called *the miracle of the Indian Ocean* by the travel industry for a period of time.

Sadly, in 2022, Sri Lanka fell in trouble again. The country accumulated an unmanageable debt, and fuel, food and electricity were short in supply. Even critical medical supplies became threatened. It was heartbreaking to see letters from children's hospitals asking for help to secure the most basic things that we took for granted in Australia. People were on the street, protesting and wanting change.

Humans make mistakes, sometimes terrible ones. It was English poet and satirist Alexander Pope who in 1711 said that 'to err is human'. But, mistakes are a learning opportunity. They help us to grow. The first step, however, is to acknowledge them. If we don't acknowledge our mistakes, we're doomed to repeat them. And like Albert Einstein said, insanity is doing the same thing over and over again and expecting a different result.

Despite seeing those traumatic scenes from the war, the memories I have of my childhood are good. My dad was an engineer for the civil service in those days. We moved around a lot because of his job; I went to around nine schools throughout my life. We lived everywhere from well-populated metropolitan centres to a small fishing town.

In the fishing town, we lived in a house that shared a plot of land with a bakery. I used to wander over in the afternoons to raid whatever delicious things were left over from the day. The sugar-filled baked goods not only tasted great, they smelled amazing. The warm, sweet smell wafting over to the house after school was my bellwether to go to the bakery. Next door was a police station. In the evenings, I jumped over the fence to hang out with the night-watch police officers who stood guard there all night. On one occasion, an officer gave me his gun to look at. Being a curious kid, I ended up firing the gun which presumably had the safety off. My parents ran out, terrified. The policeman was sacked the next day.

In this town, I went to a school that had students from a wide range of socio-economic backgrounds. There were a lot of poor kids. Some didn't even have shoes. One time, my mum bought me a pair of new shoes. They were bright white sneakers. Some of the other kids used to carry me over the water puddles because they were terrified that my new shoes would get dirty. That's how much they valued a simple thing like a new pair of shoes. To this day, I treat my shoes like those kids valued my sneakers back then. At the very least, it's out of respect for the kids like that who I know still exist on this planet.

The school was basic. Many buildings didn't have windows and were open to the elements, with only tables, chairs and a blackboard. A lot of kids lived in similar homes. The roofs were made of coconut tree branches and there was no running water or electricity. What struck me the most was the importance of education for these children. They went home from school to study by candlelight well into the night. Education was the only way they could find a better life for their families. If they graduated high school well and earned a coveted free spot at a public university, they might be able to pull their families out of poverty through a good job. Those days, many wanted a spot in a profession like medicine or engineering. Not only did those degrees secure stable jobs, but they also created migration opportunities overseas to western countries.

There was little social security. The rich–poor gap was huge. Some people quite literally had nothing; we didn't have to travel far to find beggars lining the streets.

In a town called Bandarawela that we once lived in, I went to a private school named Saint Thomas' College. The school also had another campus – its main one – in Sri Lanka's main city of Colombo. Saint Thomas' College has the second-longest uninterrupted cricket series in the world with its rival, the Royal College. Just so you know, I've been told that I'm probably the only Sri Lankan–born person in the world who is not a cricket fiend.

Saint Thomas' had proper buildings on spacious grounds. It felt serious compared to the more laid-back school of the fishing town. The socio-economic mix was different from the fishing town, too. Many parents were wealthy. It's where I was first deeply exposed to western culture thanks to two friends whose parents were doctors. I don't know what the situation is now, but at the time many doctors completed mandatory training internationally to become specialists. These particular doctors had trained in the United Kingdom. When they came back to Sri Lanka, they brought a bit of western culture back with them.

My friends played with Teenage Mutant Ninja Turtles and watched western cartoons. They ate pizza. They had video game consoles. They lived in huge houses and their parents drove European cars. One had a beautiful BMW. It was probably where my obsession with cars first developed. My friends talked about cars all the time. Their lives were totally different from what I grew up with, but I was fascinated by them. Their lifestyles inevitably rubbed off on me, as I, too, became a fan of Ninja Turtles and more importantly, pizza. But, these things weren't easily found in the country then. My parents once spent the longest time trying to find me a Ninja Turtles toy. Their quest took them to a city that was four or five hours away to find success. Pizza, too, wasn't commonplace.

Okay, I promise that this is not going to be a book about pizza.

While schools in these regional towns had some proper processes for admission, it became increasingly difficult to get a place in a school as we moved around the country. It was especially hard in some of the big population centres. Not unusually, some principals wanted a bribe. They called it a 'donation'. My mother sat outside one principal's office for days. He wouldn't see her unless the donation was paid. In the end, the only school that took me in that town was a tiny little school run out of an old house.

So, we saw war, corruption, poverty and difficulty accessing basic services. These kinds of experiences often lead people to seek a different life somewhere other than the place where they were born.

Someone who often reminds me of this is my friend Zena, who grew up in the Middle East. She experienced terrible violence there. Zena lived through times where she heard daily gunshots and bombs, which she describes as being like a whistle flying through the air followed by an explosion that shook the ground. Death was always close. She lost family members. Her family's main priority was simply to survive. They escaped by travelling through Tunisia, Jordan, Turkey, Syria and Malaysia to end up in Australia. After landing here as a refugee, she got into dental school. She studied dentistry while working two jobs. She eventually became a dentist. Imagine that. What a land of opportunity. Zena wanted to give back to that land as well. Her dream was to deliver free dental care to rural Australians. Her brother became a cardiologist. Life has become better for Zena. But, wow. What a journey to get there.

We, too, wanted a better life.

In 1994, my parents successfully applied to migrate to Australia under a skilled migration scheme. I was excited. In my short 10 years in Sri Lanka, we moved six times. Because of our transient life, I never had any meaningful connection to one place; no place had felt like home. Except for some family, there wasn't much that I was going to miss. Some of my thinking about life in Sri Lanka was shaped by the suffering I saw. I was looking forward to experiencing all the western culture that was sometimes at my fingertips but felt so far away.

We landed on the tarmac at Kingsford Smith Airport in Sydney on my 10th birthday. It was the first time I'd ever been on an aeroplane. After a few hours in the plane, airsickness gripped me. I've never vomited so much before or since. It was me, Mum, Dad and my half-sister. My half-sister didn't grow up with me in Sri Lanka, but she moved to Australia with the family.

I'll always associate Sydney with feelings of excitement and awe because it was my first taste of Australia. Even now, I have a sense of nostalgia every time I go to the city. I remember seeing the huge buildings in the CBD. I was fascinated by the Harbour Bridge, which carried so many cars in orderly lines across the water onto perfect roads extending into all parts of the city.

It was the first time I experienced the change of seasons. The summer of 1994 saw Sydney sweltering in heat. It was a very different kind of heat from Sri Lanka. The intensity was far more than the tropical heat I was used to. We lived in a red-brick apartment building in a suburb heavily populated by migrants. The building had a driveway with an open car park at the back. In the yard was a Hills Hoist that everyone shared. There was no lift, only stairs. That first summer, the Lebanese family upstairs put on Disney videos for the kids in the building. I watched *Aladdin* for the first time. They covered all the windows with dark sheets, had buckets of water around to cool face towels in and generously provided a steady supply of icy poles.

15

I'll take this opportunity to express my philosophical objection to fruit-flavoured icy poles. Or really, fruit-flavoured anything. Why not just eat the real fruit? It's my heartfelt belief that the true flavours of the world are things like chocolate and caramel, or vanilla if you are so inclined. Variations of those things are acceptable too, like salted caramel. Our household was one where the chocolate flavour was always gone in the Neapolitan ice-cream. If times became desperate, the vanilla would go too – provided there was chocolate topping around. The strawberry usually lived on till the expiry date then made it to the bin, as it should.

We didn't have much furniture initially and slept on the floor for a few days. Slowly, a charity filled our little apartment with things: old brown armchairs, a wooden single bed and a basic double bed. The four of us shared all this. We bought groceries from cavernous supermarkets. This was a novelty for me after the bustling marketplaces of Sri Lanka. What's more, the supermarkets not only had Ninja Turtles toys but all kinds of other merchandise. There was plenty of pizza everywhere. For the first time, I tasted the miracle of the lamington.

As summer drew to a close, the new school year loomed. In Sydney, I got into school through a straightforward process. No one wanted a 'donation'. We turned up one day, filled in some paperwork, and bam. I was in. The school had all kinds of children: kids with different skin colours, languages, religions and ethnicities went to school together peacefully. I have never seen such a cosmopolitan mix of people in my life. Sometimes, I caught the train to school. The slick two-tiered electric trains with an automated fare system were very different from the diesel engines of Sri Lanka that pulled overloaded cars with people hanging out the doors, the conductor yelling his way through the crowd. Differences like these gave me pause for thought about the contrasting lives that people enjoy when living in an economic power-house like Australia compared to Sri Lanka.

I made a few friends in Sydney, but no one close. Every now and again, a Vietnamese friend brought his Nintendo to my house so we could play *Mario Bros*. My mum still remembers 'that kid who came over to play Mario and farted a lot'. Video games were starting to take off then. I was quickly drawn in by games like *Mario Bros.*, *Sonic the Hedgehog* and *Mortal Kombat*. I wonder if anyone knew then, as we played those basic games, how much of a subculture video gaming would become in the years to follow. Now you know that my friend who farted a lot helped to build this culture. There actually used to be a prominent gamemaker called Gas Powered Games. I wonder if this was owned by my friend.

Just as I was starting to settle into Sydney, we moved. My dad got a job in the picturesque town of Byron Bay. It's the most easterly point on the Australian mainland, around an eight hours' drive north of Sydney. Byron Bay was a quiet little town then. Over time, though, celebrities like

Chris Hemsworth, Matt Damon and Olivia Newton-John became homeowners in the area, lifting the town's profile significantly. In the days of a small Byron Bay, I rode my bicycle to school. I played basketball and learned to play the guitar. I loved living there.

As the years went by, the dot-com bubble began to form. I was about 13 years old then, just beginning high school. I started a small business out of our garage with my mum's help. She taught me how to set up a business, a bank account, and all the other bits and pieces. I sold computers and built websites. My first big client was an importer of diving equipment whose CEO was a pilot. He had a little aircraft. In lieu of payment, I asked if he could teach me to fly in it. He agreed. Flying over the Pacific Ocean on a sunny Australian day was an indescribably beautiful thing. The world was so clear from the blue cloudless skies. I didn't fly often, but my memories of those trips are vivid.

There's a sense of serenity about flying, or, really, any activity like that. It's probably partly why I like cars too. It's you, the machine and nature. Your concentration is on operating the machine while you navigate the world in it. I find it meditative.

It was around this time that I met my high school girlfriend, Emma. Emma was a petite blonde girl with blue eyes. She was athletic and loved the band Blink-182. Apparently, she saw me dancing around on a picnic table once. I was wearing a Dallas Cowboys hat, sunglasses, tan cargo shorts and a green button-up shirt. Sexy. This was evidently an attractive enough mating dance to have piqued her interest. After a mutual friend introduced us, we became inseparable. We spent the long summers with her sitting on the handlebars of my BMX, riding around the quiet streets of Byron Bay, eating ice-cream. Magnums were our favourite. We kissed for hours on the beaches and in parks. On many Sunday afternoons, we watched the sunset bathe the valleys in gold from her dad's high-set garage roof, which was perched partway up a hill. Afterwards, she often made me nachos. Emma had a way with the nachos. I haven't tasted anything like it ever since. We talked forever on the landline phone about everything and nothing. More than once, I fell asleep with the phone on my pillow. It was good old puppy love.

The school in Byron Bay laid an important foundation for me. I went to school with a diverse cross-section of society. Some kids had rich parents. Some kids lived on welfare. Some kids had absent parents. Me, I was from a middle-class family who was yet to own a home. There was a mixture of ethnicities, religions and backgrounds. The great thing was, none of it mattered. No one cared. I never felt like an outsider. I always felt like a part of the community. I carried that through to the rest of my life. To this day, I never look at any of those things when interacting with people. I wonder if I would be different had I grown up elsewhere.

Life was pretty good for the teenage me. But inevitably, change came once more. My dad got another job. We left it all again to move to an outer-city suburb of Brisbane, four hours north of Byron Bay. As an angsty teenager, I took the move to heart. We had lived in Byron Bay for five years by that point, and it wasn't easy to leave the life that had finally become stable and happy after moving around so much. It was the longest time we had spent anywhere. Leaving Emma was painful too. But she moved on quickly – about a week later. Teenage relationships, right?

I was just finishing Year 9 when we left Byron Bay. Our new town was in another state where the kids started school at a different age. So, I jumped straight from Year 9 to Year 11. This became a point of contention in my family. Mum thought I would handle it just fine. Dad felt that I needed to go back a grade if I had any chance of doing well. Fortunately, Mum's opinion prevailed. I subsequently spent one less year in school. And for the record, Mum was right. I was challenged and grew by skipping a grade. But this is mum. She's always believed the best in me.

As the new kid in town, I was eager to make friends. I was sitting in a physics class one day when I met Daniel Wieland. I don't know why, or perhaps I can't remember, but Dan later became known as Truss. Truss was a tall guy with thick dark brown hair. In fact, he had an abundance of hair everywhere. Winter was not his enemy, for he kept naturally warm with what was effectively a built-in rug. One of our friends, who later experienced early hair loss, frequently pointed out Truss's fortunes with envy. The very first time I started talking to Truss, he asked me if I wanted to help him move a new couch that he planned to buy. Sure, I said. What better way to make a new friend than to help move furniture? That weekend, I turned up at his house and we set off on the furniture jaunt.

Truss led me to his local train station. We got into a train and stepped off a few stations later. Here was a furniture superstore. Truss handed over a couple of hundred dollars that he earned from working at a lettuce farm in exchange for an otherwise nondescript blue two-seater couch. The lettuce farm, it seemed, hadn't quite paid him enough to cover delivery. We carried the couch out of the store and onto the train, then we sat on the couch in the train until we reached Truss's home station. We got off and started walking to his house, carrying the couch on our heads. The walk was long and eventually became too laborious. Truss finally sprung for a large taxi, whose driver surprisingly agreed to stuff our couch inside by folding down the seats. Both Truss and the couch became fond friends of mine. Sadly, the couch didn't survive our trials and tribulations. Truss tells me that it died an honourable death over a decade later. Rest in peace, faithful friend.

The town was about one hour north of Brisbane. It was the cookie-cutter definition of an outer-city suburb. It had one long, straight main road lined with a shopping centre, shops, service stations and fast-food outlets. If you are familiar with Eminem's movie *8 Mile*, this is what we thought the town was like. In fact, our group of friends still call it 8 Mile. All the essentials were there. If you were inclined, there was no real need to ever leave the town. I think that many people were in fact thus inclined, spending their whole lives in 8 Mile.

There wasn't a great deal to do in 8 Mile back then. We had occasional trips to the beach, which was about half an hour away, and plenty of weekend house parties. Truss and I sometimes sat on the roof of a local medical centre at night with cans of cheap pre-mixed alcohol and just talked. The GP there had the first iteration of the Audi TT. I loved cars and always admired it. The car was a revolution in design, at least in my humble teenage opinion. The shape, the leather, the metallic switchgear – it was all beautiful.

Truss and I were both mad about cars and talked about them a lot. My favourite was the Nissan 300ZX. It was fast and had beautiful curves. It looked like a real sports car. There was a second-hand car dealer on my way to school and for the longest time, they had a black 300ZX for sale. When I walked to school, I almost always stopped to admire it. I told myself that one day I would have one.

Also in our group of friends were Jesse Richardson and the now Dr Dean McCoombe. Jesse lived with his mum, stepdad, twin brother and little sister in a big house. He loved music, Australian football and the beach. Dean grew up with his mum and his little brother. Dean knew what it was like to struggle. He came from a family with a single mum. They moved around a lot too. They had humble beginnings, making something of life with little. Dean had to grow up quickly. But he was clever and academic, and his work ethic was always strong. Through school, he always had a part-time job to keep life afloat while still getting great grades. Dean had one of those powerful minds.

Jesse was the first to get his licence and buy a car: a brown Nissan Gazelle. It had pop-up lights and I thought it was very cool. We often snuck out for McDonald's during class in Jesse's car. Each of us would in turn tell the teacher that we were going to the bathroom, meet somewhere in the school, then speed off from the car park. The teacher always raised an eyebrow when we came back to class half an hour later with McDonald's thickshakes.

Jesse picked me up for school most days, although I was often still asleep when he got to my place. Jesse was a committed friend. He was always supportive of my, what he called 'sloth-like', sleeping habits those days. He went to roll call, then skipped class to come back and pick me up. One of those days was 11 September 2001. He still remembers walking up to my door where I met him in my boxer shorts to exclaim, 'Dude, you should see what has happened in America.' It was one of those days where everyone remembers what they were doing.

Life in the suburbia of 8 Mile was uncomplicated. Mum and Dad both had local government jobs. Mum was always trying to make progress for our family. We never owned a home until then, so eventually we bought one through her persistence, a small mass-produced house in a new estate on the outskirts of 8 Mile. It was the first brand-new home that we ever lived in. We had two cars, a garden and two cats. Life was nice and comfortable. Every now and again, my maternal grandparents visited from Sri Lanka. I have good memories of eating Grandma's food after coming home from school. Sri Lankan chicken curry is delicious. The school – the ninth school I attended – was also the most interesting.

Years after I graduated from that high school, I was talking to some senior doctors about applying for specialist training programs. More than one advised, 'Put down where you finished high school in your CV, because it'll help if someone on the panel went to your school.' They assumed that I had attended a prestigious private school. When I told them the name of the public school on the outer fringes of the city that I actually went to, the instant response was, 'Oh, don't put that down.' It wasn't a school known for its academic prowess. Some of our teachers were cynical burnt-out people. Smelling like cigarettes every day, some were more interested in calling us idiots than trying to get through to us. I heard that some of my esteemed class-mates include two murderers, one person who committed grievous bodily harm, and a few others who have crossed the law for various reasons. The story is, one of them cut off someone's hands, stuffed them in the trunk of their car, then started driving to a forest to murder the victim. When they got to the forest, the victim was already dead from bleeding out. I don't know if this story is true, but this is the lore.

But, you know what? My mum likes to say that we didn't need fancy high schools to get us where we are. I agree with her. The public school education gave me insights into the world that I never would have otherwise got. It showed me the spectrum of humanity who make up a community, including the challenges that the most marginalised people face. Investing in the public school system is important, because it gives everyone an opportunity to reach for a dream no matter what their background. Critically, it taught me that no matter what environment I was in, effort can yield results. It was just up to me. Mind you, that statement feels a bit rich coming from me. I didn't always make an effort.

As a doctor, I'm sometimes asked by parents to tell their kids how hard I worked in high school. This is always uncomfortable. I know they hope that I'm going to relay a story about dedication to academics and hours of home-work, but in truth, some of my end-of-term report cards listed more than 30 days of unexplained absences. While I studied at home to get the work done, I usually left things till late. Luckily no one ever asked too many questions, because my grades were good. I just didn't find school very stimulating. I certainly didn't enjoy its structure. Often, I woke up and waited for Mum to go to work. I pretended to be getting ready for school until she left. Then, I went back to sleep and enjoyed the day. Some of my days were reminiscent of the 1986 movie *Ferris Bueller's Day Off*, even including some adventures in the family car.

I never had a particular passion when I was at school. I did a lot of fun things, but there was no purpose to them. I did well enough when I graduated high school. I ended up picking a university course that was essentially pre-dentistry. I didn't find that year super thrilling, so I started to wonder what to do next. This is where Mum came in again. By then, Mum had taught me how to drive. She taught me how to shave. She even taught me how to type. She'd shaped a great deal of who I was. And so, as my schooling neared its end, I looked to her wisdom once again to decide on a career. After much discussion, I decided to pursue a career in law. I'm sure there was a lot more thought behind why she suggested law, but for me, being a lawyer just sounded like a good job. I thought that I could make a good living, buy a house, buy a nice car, and life would be good. It was a far cry from how much I value the law today.

I applied to study law in Brisbane, and I got a spot. In 2003, I kicked off life in law school at Queensland University of Technology. Although I was excited to fly out into the world, I didn't realise that the world was about to fling me into the darkness.

2

THE BLACK DOG

You should think of the word 'depressed' as 'deep rest.'
Your body needs to be depressed. It needs deep rest from
the character that you've been trying to play.

Jim Carrey

ALTHOUGH I FIND it interesting now, reading law at university wasn't always exciting. The thick tax and constitutional law books made for dry reading. Often, those books of mine were still in mint condition at the end of the semester. Untouched, still shrink-wrapped.

I wasn't growing a love for the law. Instead, I spent a lot of time amusing myself with things like a pretty girlfriend, my fast car – a black Nissan 300ZX finally – and nightlife. I quickly got caught up in a superficial world, drawn in by the trappings of society.

I remember sitting in a lecture once with a guy and a girl. The guy had a Louis Vuitton bag. The girl was teasing him about it being fake. I didn't even know what a Louis Vuitton bag was at that point. In Sri Lanka, one of these bags would be worth well over the annual average national salary, maybe even a few times over. I never saw one in 8 Mile either. They proceeded to talk about Louis Vuitton bags, which then deteriorated into an argument about whether Mercedes was better than BMW. The conversation wasn't in friendly jest, but in poisonous barbs designed to put each other down. In their eyes, the deepest insult was to imply that the other had a lower level of wealth or that their taste in luxury goods was ridiculous.

One of my girlfriends enjoyed the material side of life as well. She loved anything that the latest gossip magazine socialite was into. Her dream was simply to be famous. I think that when you don't have a well-developed sense of self, it's natural to follow the flow of the people around you. You become shaped by them. That was me. My goals became superficial too. I started thinking about earning lots of money. I wanted nice things. I wanted to become a partner in a big law firm so I could buy those things.

Eckhart Tolle said, 'The most common ego identifications have to do with possessions, the work you do, social status and recognition, knowledge and education, physical appearance, special abilities, relationships, personal and family history, belief systems, and often also political, nationalistic, racial, religious, and other collective identifications. None of these is you.' I didn't know the real me but was misguidedly trying to find an identity in some of those things. I didn't realise that I was sinking deeper and deeper into unhappiness as a result. There was a slow-growing dark cloud above me that I didn't see until it was too late.

I did make a couple of friends in law school. I met James Mourdhuj in one of the introductory law classes. In contrast to the thick lush follicles commanded by Truss, I've never known Jimmy to have hair. He had a similar skin colour to mine and was nearly the same height. Jimmy became a partner in crime who I often studied with. We bonded over our commonalities – we both liked hip-hop and skipped class to eat at our favourite Indian restaurant. Twelve dollars bought two curries, some naan bread, rice and a drink, although the heavy Indian meal usually put us to sleep rather than fuel us for study. We were profound procrastinators whose assignments were routinely finished during last-minute all-nighters.

Once, Jimmy and I were so sleepy after being in the library all night that on the drive home, being responsible budding lawyers, we decided to pull over at a park to sleep. My 300ZX only had two seats. Jimmy took off his shirt in the summer heat and slept in the front. I opened the shallow boot and laid down, settling into as comfortable a position as I could manage. One of my legs was hanging out of the boot. We both fell into a deep sleep.

Some time later, I opened my eyes to see a police officer standing over me.

'Uhhh . . . hello.'

'Someone reported two dead bodies in a car,' she said.

'Oh. Well, we're both alive.'

'That's good. It's less paperwork for us,' she said.

After a breath alcohol test, we were set free.

When I was at university, I had a job at McDonald's. I worked there with Jesse and Daniel. We cooked burgers in the back while playing hip-hop on a boombox, checking out the cute girl customers through the gap in the burger warmer. At the start, I was paid $6 per hour or thereabouts. After an entire week's work, the paycheque was around $300. For a while, I worked in a 24-hour McDonald's as well. Sometimes, I did night shifts, then went to class in the morning smelling like grease.

The reality is, I didn't have to do any of that because my parents looked after me well. But, I wanted to learn some life skills. And I did. There was no better place to learn the importance of things like systems than McDonald's. Their systems were set up so I could make 12 cheeseburgers in two and a half minutes. It was a well-oiled machine.

After McDonald's, I worked in the video game section at Harvey Norman. I was a terrible salesman. I gave most people a discount, even when they didn't ask for one. That was the job that took me through to the latter part of law school.

Law school was a competitive place, at times ruthlessly so. I once did a small tax law assignment but didn't go to the class to hand it in. I entrusted it to a colleague. When I got a zero for the assignment, I queried this with the tutor. He told me that I never handed the assignment in. It turned out my colleague had copied the assignment verbatim, handed it in as his own and thrown mine out. The amazing thing is, when I asked him about it, he told me exactly what he had done with a perfectly straight, unsurprised face. It was as if I had asked a silly question. Many years later, the same colleague fell under scrutiny by the authorities for questionable practices. I guess old habits die hard for some.

A more important point is the reason why I didn't go to that tax tutorial. By then, that dark cloud had mushroomed to envelope my entire sky. I was struggling with depression, anxiety, panic attacks and agoraphobia – the fear of leaving a safe environment because of a potential panic attack. It was something that I had never experienced before. Things were so bad sometimes that I was afraid to go outside the house. That's what happened that day. That's why I gave my friend the assignment to hand in. I was too afraid to go to the class.

These conditions caused physical symptoms that seemed so real. When I had panic attacks, I felt short of breath. Sometimes, I had palpitations. I felt an unspecified sense of doom, as though something terrible was going to happen. I felt that maybe I was going to die imminently. Maybe the universe was going to collapse on itself. Maybe I was going to have a heart attack.

Depression disturbed my sleep cycles. I was waking up at about 3 am with no alarm. Then, I couldn't sleep again.

My appetite changed. The anxiety was bad, and it was there all the time. I was heightened constantly. I felt constantly on the edge, like I was in a war zone. The smallest thing set me off – a sound, a sensation, a light. Being hypervigilant all the time was exhausting.

It was a combination of these things that gave me agoraphobia. For weeks, I thought that only my house was safe. I was inside all the time. Even stepping out into the garden caused me to panic.

When I wasn't in a state of panic or anxiety, I didn't feel anything. I was flat. I was sad. I didn't taste the food. I didn't hear the music. I didn't see the light. I didn't feel the sun on my skin. The world was grey. I felt like a human being alone in an apocalyptic world, with no hope in sight.

A friend in law school tried to help me through it. One day, we arranged to meet up for a chat, but I was too scared to leave the house and I cancelled. My friend became very frustrated. He snapped, 'You need to go sit in a park and think about your life.' I understand how this frustration can creep in when people are trying to reach out to you and you won't – or can't – engage with them. It's easy to think that someone isn't trying to help themselves when that happens, but in reality they're just trapped within their thoughts. Depression is an isolating thing that way. When I continued to reject my friends' help, the people around me lost patience and I became even more alone. It was a self-perpetuating black hole.

I've now had the benefit of dealing with both depression and physical paralysis. I can tell you right now that depression paralysed me more than the spinal cord injury ever has. I know this is a big claim to make. Still, I firmly believe that being a prisoner of the mind is far more debilitating than any limit of the body. Stephen Hawking is a great example. His body was completely locked, but his mind was powerful. He changed the way humanity views the universe. When the mind is free, the universe opens.

When I was depressed, I wasn't productive in any sense of the word. My relationships suffered. Work suffered. Education suffered. It was utterly debilitating. Paradoxically, since physical paralysis, I've achieved more in my life than I ever had before. I wouldn't wish either challenge on anyone, but I find this a fascinating comparison. It's why we need to understand mental health issues better and find better ways to treat them.

This was one of the most difficult periods in my life. But, it turned out to be one of the best things that ever happened to me.

One manifestation of depression or anxiety can be a preoccupation with death. I thought about death a lot. In turn, I thought about life as well. Most importantly, I thought about what my life might look like in retrospect at the time of my death. I started to think about what would make me feel like I had lived a worthy life.

Over the years, I've had many chances to reflect not

just on what a worthy life is, but on its uncertainty. Life is not eternal, at least in the way in which you and I are experiencing it right now. We don't know when the candle will be extinguished.

In fact, this is a principle of Stoicism. *Memento mori*, as they call it, is a reminder to reflect on our mortality. On this, Marcus Aurelius the stoic philosopher king said to 'let each thing you would do, say, or intend, be like that of a dying person'. So, *memento mori* helps us clear the meaningless things within our beings, to prioritise what is most important to us. It's not a meditation on death itself, but on how to live best.

I have a friend who has Huntington's disease. Statistically, they know that they have about 10 years before the symptoms of the disease will develop – around the age of 40. It's a progressive genetic condition that will eventually take their cognitive, physical and emotional faculties.

Ten years. My friend is counting on 10 years of good life. When I spend time with them, the value of life becomes so apparent. We often talk about things like love, which is unique for both of us because of our situations. For my friend, because their life will inevitably change into something so different within a limited time. For me, because it already has. Every day, my friend is deeply aware of the urgent need to make the most of their life before things change. Unsurprisingly, the things that they have prioritised are not ones like a career or the accumulation of objects.

They are meaningful things like memories, love and family. Even though it's very pronounced for my friend, we might all do well to consider life in this way.

And, you know, many of us mightn't even have 10 years. How many people have woken up in the morning, then had a fatal accident? A stroke? A heart attack? Sadly, working as a doctor, I see people like this all the time. I wonder how many of them realised that it was going to be their last day on earth.

Memento mori.

How do we make the most of life in the limited time we have? I think above all, we need to spend our days doing things that are meaningful to us. In my journey through depression, I found something that felt meaningful to me.

When I was recovering from depression, I began to interact with doctors. Once I started to get better, I realised that their help had changed my world. I was incapacitated before then, but with help, I became a functioning human being again. What's more, my grey world started to change. I saw colours again. I tasted the food. The music sounded melodic. The sun, oh, the sun – it felt so good on my skin. I remember the day, the very instant, I realised that my world was transformed. It was a moment when I drove out of the garage and suddenly felt the visceral experience of this beautiful world. It went from being a barren wasteland to unbridled paradise. I was connected to it. And I realised, I'm alive again.

My mum loves ᐧto quote the saying, 'By helping one person, you may not change the world – but you will change the world for them.' This philosophy resonated deeply with me. After a great deal of thought, I decided that I wanted to be a doctor too. Imagine, every day my job would be potentially changing someone's world for the better. Here was a career where I could use my head and my heart to help anyone, anywhere. There was a purity to that idea. It would be intellectually challenging too. I could continually learn, grow. I knew that to me, this would be a life well lived. But if I'm honest, it was the TV show *Grey's Anatomy* that sealed the deal. Those doctors were getting all the girls.

Through finding myself, I found purpose. The search for who we are is different for each one of us. Some of us know who we are from the moment we are born. Some of us spend years being wandering souls who the world eventually nudges – or, as in my case, forces – to the right place. For all of us, the purpose is different. Some of us come alive by creating art. Some of us are energised by building things. Some of us run. Some of us explore. Some of us become healers. It's when we find the purpose that resonates with our real self, that light shines to brighten our world. Then, we truly begin to live.

This is the trick, my friends. To find ourselves and reveal our purpose. That is how I decided to become a doctor.

My decision was timely, because my schoolfriend Dean decided to study medicine too. He was working as a radiographer then. Radiographers are the people who take X-rays, CT scans and MRIs. He had a natural gift for the sciences and had always been a clever guy. We started chasing the dream together. It was like being back in school.

The path to medical school involved three phases. First, we had to have at least an undergraduate degree in something. That something could be anything, although something in the sciences was helpful. The results from that degree needed to be decent. Second, we needed a competitive result in the medical school entrance exam. This was a five-and-a-half-hour exam heavily weighted towards sciences. Essay writing was a component as well. Thirdly and finally, we needed to perform well in an interview.

Never had I been more motivated to achieve results. I felt energised. I felt alive. I had purpose. Gone were the days of lethargy and procrastination. I busted my butt to bring my law degree marks up because unsurprisingly, after my depressive journey, they weren't great. I worked much harder from then on, because I had a dream.

Dean and I started studying for the entrance exam. After not doing any science since high school, I was rusty, so I did some courses and saw a tutor every week. Let me tell you right now, I didn't enjoy chemistry. I had no interest in learning about carbon chains or organic molecules, but I did it anyway to work towards the greater good. I liked physics, though. It just made sense to me. Today, I don't remember much of what we learned then. I don't spend a great deal of time thinking about the structure of molecules while trying to diagnose a heart attack.

I went to Dean's house every couple of days. We talked through the science books and practised an endless number of questions. I aggressively raided Dean's fridge. It really bothered his then girlfriend. Every time I went to the fridge to find a snack, she magically appeared with a stern face to ask me what I was doing.

Dean got into medical school a year before me, because he finished his undergraduate degree earlier than me. A year later, I sat the entrance exam. I had food poisoning that day. Maybe that was the universe punishing me for raiding Dean's fridge. I slept in the car in between papers and went home thinking that I had done terribly. Months later, I got the result. It was competitive enough to get into medical school.

I sat the interview. The interview included a scenario about an airport that had a sudden unexpected significant influx of passengers. The interview panel asked me various questions about the situation. What might have caused it? What might be some solutions? Could I explain it on the whiteboard in front of me? They were sizing up my ability to reason, analyse, and explain things. They then asked the standard questions, like why I wanted to be a doctor.

Prospective medical students often ask me what the right answer to this question is. There's a thought among some that wanting to help people is the wrong answer. They say that it's too standard. It's too boring. It's the answer I gave.

In my opinion, it's the most important and relevant answer to the question. If you don't want to help people, you probably need to rethink your reasons for becoming a doctor.

A short time after the interview, I received an email offering me a place with a scholarship. My university fees were to be paid and I'd get a stipend to study medicine. I printed the offer, folded it, then gave it to Mum, saying that it was a speeding ticket that needed to be paid. The look on her face when she saw what it really contained was priceless.

I started medical school in Queensland's Griffith University in 2008. I moved in with Dean and we lived in an apartment overlooking the ocean in the Gold Coast. We shared a large fridge with no girlfriend as a sentry. Dean was now single so I could raid it any time without fear of any fierce looks. From day one of medical school, I knew that I realised my purpose. I loved medicine. Life was good.

We were a class of about 120 students, mostly in our early to mid-20s. I was 23. Many had a background in science. A few others, like me, came from diverse academic backgrounds like law. We even had a music therapist who eventually became a surgeon. Initially, I felt like a bit of an outsider. Actually, I felt pretty stupid most of the time. Many of my classmates were well versed in basic physiology and other relevant sciences. I had no idea. I spent a lot of time learning the basics in order to come up to speed. After about six months, I finally felt like I caught up enough to be at the same level as everyone else.

The first two years of medical school were spent in class. It was different from most degrees in that there weren't subjects in the classical sense. Rather, there were blocks where we learned about different body systems. We learned the normal function of a system like the respiratory or cardiovascular systems, and then the abnormal function – diseases. Pharmacology, ethics, law, epidemiology and physical examination were all strategically embedded in those blocks. The course didn't follow standard semesters, either. This unique format was a necessity due to the nature of medicine and its voluminous content. As those two years progressed, we gradually started venturing into the hospital.

The pressure to keep up was significant. If you failed a year, you repeated the entire year. There was a limit to the number of those repeats. If you reached that limit, the next step was exclusion.

Through the challenges of medical school, we all became close. Everyone knew each other's names. We cared about each other. We studied hard, but blew off steam just as hard. Friday afternoon gatherings were plentiful. There was a pub a short walk from the medical school. We gathered there, bought buckets of Coronas, then debriefed on the events of the week.

I met a woman, too. I'll call her Yaris. She was a motivated student. Yaris stayed with me and Dean some nights, because her home was an hour's drive away. While we played video games, *Grand Theft Auto* mostly, Yaris studied. She loved to cook. We were well fed when she stayed. We were friends first, but eventually started dating. Yaris was thoughtful and generous, but sadly, things didn't work out and we broke up after a couple of months.

The first two years of medical school went by, culminating in halfway celebrations. The final two years of medical school were going to be even more exciting because we would be located nearly fulltime in hospitals. We were to rotate through specialties like emergency medicine, internal medicine, obstetrics and gynaecology, anaesthetics, and surgery. Our time was focused on the practical preparation to be a doctor. My first rotation was in psychiatry.

My supervisor was Professor Harry McConnell. Harry grew up in America and went to university at McGill in Canada. McGill has a special reputation for science and a history of alumni like Ernest Rutherford who developed the eponymous model of the atom. Fostered by that environment, Harry had an impressive intellect. He retained his American accent. To me, he was a mixture of Robin Williams and Mel Gibson. If those two people had a baby, it would be Harry. He was not only clever but passionate about helping marginalised people. I didn't know then how big a role his passion would play later in my journey.

Just before I started psychiatry, I took a spur-of-the-moment trip to Japan with my close medical school friend, Daniel Gillespie. Dan was from a country town and both his parents were GPs. They also farmed wagyu beef, so Dan often had a good supply of steak. He used to study at my place for exams and in the evenings, barbecued us the perfect steak. A few weeks before third year started, Dan asked me if I wanted to go to Japan. I thought about the idea for a while, and almost said no in order to save my pennies and study, but ultimately I decided to go. We packed one bag each and turned up in Tokyo without any plans. On a whim, we made our way by train to Niseko, over a thousand kilometres to the north. It was the second time in my life that I saw snow. It was beautiful, like something from a Disney movie. Taking that trip with Dan taught me something: *Carpe diem*. Seize the day.

We intellectualise some decisions so much, don't we? Whether it be because of time, money, what someone else thinks, work or whatever, we overthink things. We miss out on so much life as a result. As we become adults, spontaneity diminishes. We think about the future, and sometimes rightly so. Responsibilities weigh on us. Kids come along. The mortgage looms. But in the thick of it all, time keeps ticking with no certainty about what the future will bring. There's the fear of the unknown too, but I like to think that we are far happier reaching into the unknown than having regrets about not trying. When I reminisce with Dan now, we don't talk about how much money we could've saved. Hell, we don't even talk about our grades. We talk about one of the greatest trips ever.

I wonder how much less I would've hesitated to take that trip too if someone had told me that I would never stand in the snow atop a mountain like that again, feeling snowflakes falling onto my face on a silent winter's evening. I wonder how much more I would've savoured that time while I was away. There's so much truth in the thought that what matters most is the moment that we have right in front of us. It's a gift. One to be grateful for. One to squeeze every drop out of.

When we came back, medical school kicked off again. Things were a little different. I put the shorts and t-shirt away in exchange for clinically presentable clothes. My psychiatry rotation was located at a private psychiatric hospital in a pleasant neighbourhood just a block away from the beach in southern Gold Coast. The days there were good. We spent the morning seeing patients, then wandered over to the beach for lunch. The afternoon was a mixture of things, but mostly slow paced.

We had the occasional lecture back at the medical school on a variety of topics. But, I remember one really well. It was a lecture given by an emergency physician, Dr Stephen Rashford. Dr Rashford worked for the ambulance service. He talked about the pointy end of medicine. There were photos of extreme trauma, of him performing lifesaving interventions. I remember seeing my place in those photos, thinking it this was something that I'd love to do. It sparked an early interest in trauma and emergency medicine.

On weekends, I frequently visited my parents who still lived in 8 Mile. They lived about an hour and a half away from me. One visit occurred on a weekend in late January 2010. My half-sister flew in from Canberra with her new-ish boyfriend, and I wanted to say hello to her. I always liked being home and eating Mum's food anyway. It was a good weekend full of family, laughter and happiness. Sunday came all too quickly. I planned to leave early that day, but the vibe at my parents' home was so relaxed that I lazed around the house till late. Then, I decided stay for dinner. Mum, of course, was all too pleased to have this extra time with me, even if my activity consisted mainly of lying about and eating chicken curry.

After dinner, I finally gathered myself to leave. I gave my mum a hug and stepped into my 2004 silver Nissan X-Trail. This was the last thing I ever did standing up. To this day, I love being able to say that the last thing I did while standing up was hug my mum.

I drove out to the highway. It was a crisp night after intermittent rain throughout the day. The air smelt fresh. The road looked sharp under the lights. I was driving just under the speed limit because of the wet road and listening to some old rap. I like all music, but have a penchant for old rap. I grew up with Tupac, but later grew to like Biggie. Tupac was a little dark. He was deep. Biggie was happy. His music fit that time of my life, because I too was happy. In fact, life was perfect.

Sometimes, I can't help but think of destiny. Here we are, in the infinite expanse of the universe. Is it really just by chance that you and I are now sharing this conversation after evolving from a primordial soup, millions of years ago? Possibly, but what an incomprehensible concept that is to toss about in one's mind. Either way, whether through chance or destiny, I ended up on a particular stretch of highway on the night of 31 January 2010. It was a little messy from recent roadworks. I drove through it, still relaxed. Suddenly, I saw a shiny black slick up ahead in my lane. It was too late to avoid it.

The moment I hit it, my car lost control and started spinning around. My body responded before my brain did. Adrenaline surged through my bloodstream. I thought I regained control for a second – a fleeting chance of reprieve, perhaps. No. The car spun off again. It mounted a roadside embankment. As it descended back towards the road, the nose struck the tarmac. The vehicle flew through the air, nose to tail.

Inside the car was unbridled destruction. Things were flying around the cabin: my laptop, my phone, my bags. I heard glass explode and shatter. Every time the car bounced on the road, violent metallic sounds pierced the tranquil night air. In between the cacophony were moments of silence – almost of stillness – while the car was intermittently airborne.

At this point, I realised that there was nothing I could do to stop what was happening.

Although I didn't know what it was then, there's a great technique called *cognitive reframing* which enables us to view negative situations differently. For example, you change the thought 'this is too hard' to 'I love a challenge'.

As the accident was happening, I decided to frame it as something different. I chose not to view it as something scary. Instead, I decided to think of it as a roller-coaster. I'll have fun, I thought. And so, I whooped through the car crash like a guy riding the world's best roller-coaster. There it is. Emotional wellbeing techniques in action through one of the most chaotic moments in my life.

The car landed after what seemed like an eternity. It was dead silent except for the occasional creak and hiss. I looked around. The car was destroyed. I looked down. My white t-shirt was soaked in blood. I felt no pain. I felt no fear either, until I tried to get out. I couldn't move. My fingers didn't work. I couldn't grab the door handle. I put that hand on my leg. I couldn't feel it.

Oh God.

Have you ever been in a situation where something un-imaginably bad happens in an instant? Do you remember the horror? I can't begin to explain what I felt when I realised what happened. My soul suffocated. A thousand thoughts raced through my mind. In those seconds, my life changed forever. It was never to be the same again.

Carpe diem. This is why.

The car behind me pulled over. Driving it was a guy

named Chris Bailey. I didn't meet Chris properly until five years later, but he ran up, reached through the driver's side window and checked on me. He knew that I was badly hurt. He held my head, because my neck was apparently floppy at that stage. He got blood all over him. He didn't have a phone, so another car passing by called emergency services.

A fire truck was the first emergency vehicle to turn up. Chris was annoyed because he thought it drove right past us. But in reality, the driver had lost control like I had after running over the oil slick or whatever it was on the road, and the truck slid right past my car. They reversed back. I was cut out of the car with the jaws of life and put in an ambulance which had arrived by then. This was the start of my journey as a patient.

I looked up in the ambulance and was surprised to see Dr Stephen Rashford. 'You lectured me not long ago,' I said. We connected silently for a moment, him realising that I was a medical student. I felt okay for a minute in the presence of a familiar face. Then, I became distressed again. The horror came over me again. How would I become a doctor? How would I live? I was terrified.

Dr Rashford taught me something else that night. And for me, that moment crystallised what being a doctor is fundamentally about.

In the halls of the emergency department of the Gold Coast University Hospital hangs a big photo of Dr Leo Marneros. The late Dr Marneros was an emergency physician. Sadly I never met him, but his humanism is famed. I'm told that he loved the saying inspired by Maya Angelou, 'More than what you do for them, people will remember how you made them feel.'

This is what I learned in the ambulance on that fateful night.

I knew that Dr Rashford was a skilled physician. Yet, his technical performance is not what I remember years later. It's what he said to me in that moment of distress. 'We're taking you to the best hospital for these injuries,' he said. 'Everything will be okay. If you want to get back to medicine after this, you'll find a way.' I remember how he made me feel. I felt at ease again. At least, as at ease as I could be under the circumstances.

In the firestorm that I was suddenly thrown into, though, I had no idea what was to come.

3

THE DARKEST TIMES, THE HARDEST DAYS

In the meantime, cling tooth and nail to the following rule: not to give in to adversity, not to trust prosperity, and always take full note of fortune's habit of behaving just as she pleases.

Seneca

THE NEXT THING I remember was being in a hospital bed. It was cold. I couldn't feel my body. I couldn't move. It was like my body was chopped off completely below the chest. You know the way in magic shows, when the assistant is in a box, sawn in half, with their torso and legs seemingly completely disconnected from their head? That was how I felt.

Bright white clinical lights burned into my eyes. Something weird was attached to my head. I realised that it was traction – a way of attempting to pull my spine back into place. To do this, two screws were secured into my head with a contraption attached to some weights. I still have the scars from the screws. The idea was for the weight to pull the dislocated spine back into place. I felt a bit calmer at this point, but the reality of what had happened was still sinking in.

Mum walked in. Her face was expressionless and I knew that she was worried. Apparently, she was told the worst-case scenario – that I mightn't survive; that I might never breathe on my own; that I might never be able to lift my arms up. She was told that if I survived, I might be in a vegetative state – that is, completely unresponsive.

I hated seeing my mum sad. There's nothing more painful to me. In that moment, I knew what she was feeling. I wanted her to feel okay. It was one of those times where your love for someone overtakes your own distress. So I said, 'I'm okay, Mum. Everything is going to be okay.' Years later, Mum told me that as soon as I said those words, she knew that everything truly would be okay.

There's nothing in the universe like the love of a mother. When a child is in pain, their mother feels pain too. I've seen it. I've heard it. More than once, parents have tragically lost their children in our emergency department. I'll never forget their cries. It's heart-wrenching.

There's a story I heard about a mother whose son sustained a severe brain injury when he was very young. He was in a vegetative state for years. Every day, the mother tended to him. She talked to him. She hoped that he would wake up. The last I heard, 10 years had passed. The mother was still by her son's side every day, talking to him, hoping that he would wake up. That's love.

I met another mother whose son also had a brain injury. She always wanted him to improve. To understand the brain better, she did a psychology degree. Then, she worked on a clinical trial looking at improving brain function in people with those injuries. 'I won't give up,' she said to me. She promised to find a way. There was so much conviction in her voice. That's love.

Tell me, where else in the universe do you find this kind of dedication from one person to another?

I don't know how long I was in traction for. But it didn't work. Within hours, the doctors looking after me made a decision to take me into the operating theatre. My spine had to be surgically fixed. As I was being wheeled there, I asked someone who was presumably the anaesthetist what was happening to me. He said something like, 'You're very badly injured. I can't guarantee that you'll wake up from this.' While I don't remember his exact words, I remember how he made me feel too – terrified. I felt distressed again. Soon, I fell asleep.

In an article called 'Little white lies in the resus room', Dr Simon Carley writes about this point in time during a resuscitation – when the patient becomes unconscious, and a breathing tube goes down into their throat. In the piece,

Dr Carley describes a hypothetical patient named John: 'I know, you know, and everyone else in the room knows that this is a life threatening injury. We all know that that John will probably not survive and that the next 10 minutes might well be the last conscious moments of his life.

'What do I say to John?' he concludes.

He wonders, do you tell a white lie and say that everything will be okay? Otherwise, do you tell them that this is a critical injury so they at least have an opportunity to say goodbye to their family? In among the controlled chaos and technical things happening in a resuscitation room, these are the deeply human issues that can make an impact.

On the technical side, I never really thought about what happened behind the scenes medically in the initial stages after the accident. Later though, I thought a lot about it after taking a course on how to better manage trauma – serious injuries – in the emergency department. It was the first time this course had had a participating doctor using a wheelchair. While I've been involved with trauma patients at work, the course gave me a better insight into the mechanics of trauma resuscitation in an emergency department. I now realise that I would've gone through a well-orchestrated process when the accident happened.

The first phase in trauma is prehospital management. This refers to the treatments that are given to the patient before they even get to hospital. It's vital that no time is wasted on activity that does not add value to the care of the patient. So sometimes, paramedics 'scoop and run', where the patient is rushed to hospital urgently, lights flashing and sirens blaring. The patient may have some treatment en route. At other times, paramedics 'stay and play' at the scene, conducting treatment that's time-critical and cannot wait until transport to hospital.

In metropolitan centres, this is usually a relatively smooth process. Hospitals are close and those hospitals have every specialty and piece of equipment on hand. Patients who have serious trauma can get to a hospital within an hour.

It's a different story in rural areas. Some places don't have ambulances. It's not unusual to hear stories about people who've been lying on the side of the road for hours, injured, in pain and in fear, waiting for help. I know a guy with a spinal cord injury who experienced just that after a motorbike accident. He lay in a ditch paralysed for many hours until someone found him.

Some places don't have a hospital. Some have a small hospital with one exhausted doctor. Most injured patients will need to be flown to a large hospital that can handle complex trauma. The patient will be away from their family for a long time. More importantly, life-threatening injuries or illnesses may only be temporarily stabilised until they get somewhere. These temporary measures are not always guaranteed to last.

The rural–metropolitan inequity is a fascinating contrast. Where I live and work, our patients have access to rapid lifesaving care in a state-of-the-art hospital. If they have a stroke or heart attack, a patient has access to a life-sustaining procedure within an hour. For someone living rurally, it can take days – or at times they may never get to the needed interventions. Even in geographically small countries like Sri Lanka, this is still the case. Metropolitan areas are far better resourced. Having said that, doctors who work in rural areas have the opportunity to make a huge impact and do impressive medicine with very little resources. I often think that rural doctors practice the purest form of medicine – it's just them and the patient.

When paramedics can get to a patient, there are a lot of things they can do when they 'stay and play'. The most extreme procedure in emergency management of trauma by an appropriately skilled person is to crack open someone's chest. If the patient is on the verge of death because of certain carefully recognised serious injuries inside the chest, this is the last-ditch, nothing-to-lose procedure that may have a slim chance of saving a life that's otherwise slipping away. There are scattered stories of colleagues doing the procedure at the roadside.

Once a patient is stabilised and transport begins, a hospital is notified. In some hospitals, this is through what is fondly called the *Bat Phone*. In the large hospital that I work in, once notified of the imminent arrival of an injured patient, a 'trauma alert' or 'trauma respond' page is triggered. A trauma alert means that something serious has happened, but the injuries may not be too severe. In these cases, a core team is ready in the resuscitation room with other specialties on stand-by if needed. If it's a trauma respond, everyone will rush to the resuscitation room. This'll include people like surgeons, intensive care specialists and anaesthetists. Sometimes, the room can be full of doctors, nurses and other personnel. Someone will generally conduct some crowd control and 'decant' the room to keep only the most useful people inside. You probably don't need the wandering urologist for the head trauma patient. Well, I guess you might for a special class of people who could have urological trauma on the head. We all know some, don't we?

The core medical team consists of a team leader, airway doctor, assessment doctor and procedure doctor. A core nursing team will be present as well. They, too, will be assigned specific roles. There'll also be a radiographer to take X-rays, a scribe to note everything down, and other staff depending on what's happening at that time.

The job of the team leader is to orchestrate all the moving parts in the room. Their role is to have a bird's-eye view of everything and direct the management of the patient. The airway doctor has one important job: to manage the patient's airway. If the airway is lost, everything is lost – the patient dies. This is a critical task which requires a great deal of skill and concentration. The airway doctor is also responsible for assessing any head and neck injuries, as they are positioned at the head of the bed.

The assessment doctor will work from below the head. They'll assess for any bodily injuries and perform activities like bedside ultrasounds. The procedure doctor will insert lines, chest tubes, and perform other procedures as needed. It can be chaotic. But, a skilled trauma team can manage the chaos calmly. Hopefully, they keep the patient alive in the face of any injury that threatens life.

A similar team would have been activated to manage my trauma. There must have been an airway doctor, perhaps someone who protected my neck; a procedure doctor might have inserted an intravenous line or two; someone might have inserted a catheter into my bladder.

Once they stabilised me and after the traction failed, I went to the operating theatre. There, my throat was opened up to access the spine from the front. The spine was then put back into place and secured by two screws. The surgeons took some bone from my hip, then grafted it to my spine to secure it even more. Despite the scepticism of the anaesthetist, I made it to the intensive care unit alive.

Over the next three days or so, I started to open my eyes. Everything was blurry. I felt the tube down my throat pushing air into my lungs. I could make out people in the room. The first person I saw was a guy who I went to medical school with. I'll call him Angus. 'Ah, there he is,' he said with a smile.

Some time later, I was finally extubated. That is, the breathing tube was taken out. Breathing for myself was still difficult. I woke up properly and started crying. Mum came in. 'I'm crippled,' I cried out.

The weight of what had happened choked me. I don't know how else to explain it. I felt it in my chest. I felt it in my throat. I felt it in my soul. I couldn't stop thinking about it.

The ICU was a difficult environment. I had tubes everywhere. I had a tube going near the heart to deliver drugs. I also had a tube coming out of my neck. That's where the spinal surgery was conducted. The tube was attached to a ball-shaped container. The container filled slowly with blood, the only evidence of the passage of time. I didn't know whether it was night or day.

I started to hallucinate after a while. In one hallucination, I floated up through the floor above, which was now a chessboard. I became a piece on that chessboard. Other pieces were trying to kill me. I was the king they were aiming to check. It was terrifying.

Although I drifted in and out of consciousness, I found it almost impossible to sleep. A million thoughts were rushing through my head. One night, I wanted to be put to sleep so I begged for some midazolam – an effective sedative. They finally gave me something which put me to sleep for a short while.

The days rolled on. When the evenings came, everyone went home and I was alone with the ICU nurse. They sat at the entrance to my room, with a computer screen lighting up their face. It was eerie. I was alone with my thoughts. The realisation that I was paralysed kept coming to me like a sledgehammer pounding away at a crumbling rock. *I am paralysed. Life will never be the same again.* It was sickening. The thought was so strong that it overshadowed anything else that I tried to think about. I didn't want to be with my thoughts. I begged for a distraction. After searching the hospital, the staff were able to get a TV and DVD player into my room. One of the first movies I watched while in intensive care was Spielberg's *Minority Report*. I probably should have picked something less atmospheric and more lighthearted. Every time I see *Minority Report* now, I'm instantly taken back to the ICU. The memory is hardwired into the core of my being.

In the thick of one of those nights, I was lying there, again unable to sleep. A doctor walked into the room to do some perfunctory tasks like checking observations and recharting medications. He didn't say a word to me. I broke the silence and asked him about my prognosis. It was all I could think about. Against the odds, I was wishing for someone to tell me that I'll get up and walk. For some reason, the doctor became incredibly annoyed. 'Hasn't someone explained what's going on already?' he snapped before storming out of the room. To this day, I don't understand why he responded that way.

There's a lot of inexplicable behaviour in medicine. As a medical student, I came across one doctor who was as brash as they come. We were doing a ward round one morning. Under our care was a generously built person who probably wasn't going to live too long because of a rapidly deteriorating medical condition. That day, when we walked in, this patient asked, 'Why is this happening to me?' The doctor responded bluntly, 'It's because you're fat,' before we all marched out of the room. Sadly, I can tell you quite a few of these stories.

It's important to have the right people in medicine. Otherwise, patients can sustain serious damage – injuries far deeper than the ones they came into hospital with. Some people get into the profession for reasons that are inconsistent with a job so fundamentally rooted in caring for humans. Some become arrogant over time. Some forget why we chose this job. For some, it's just that – a job. I don't think medicine can ever truly be just a job. At the centre of it is a human being. In fact, two human beings – the one being cared for and the one doing the caring. In that dynamic, there has to be a love for the human you are caring for. Hippocrates is said to have noted, 'Wherever the art of medicine is loved there is also a love of humanity.' That can't be truer.

I once attended a medical conference in San Francisco. In the room for one session were patients and doctors together. The patients were asked to explain what they wanted most from their care. The doctors were asked to respond. What happened was fascinating. The room erupted into a heated argument. The patients wanted the doctors to enable them to live their ideal life, despite a medical condition. The doctors said that their job was only to fix the medical problem the best they can.

Sadly, some patients went on to say that they have a version of post-traumatic stress from regularly attending hospitals for chronic medical problems.

I can relate to this. My experience of being in hospital was terrible.

I won't go to a hospital today as a patient unless I'm dying. I work in a hospital nearly every day. I love being a doctor, but I hate being a patient. Because of that reflection, I'm mindful of how much we can build or destroy the therapeutic relationship between doctor and patient by our actions, big or small.

My experiences inform the way I practise medicine today. When I see patients, I remember what I went through. I can guess what they must be feeling because I felt it too. In my practice, I try to be just as much a human as I am a doctor. Just as Hippocrates talked about the love of humanity, Plato said that 'no attempt should be made to cure the body without the soul'. He said that the greatest error physicians make is to separate the soul from the body. I know how true that observation is.

In the ICU, I learned to let go of everything, starting with my dignity. I was naked all the time, partly because clothing predisposed me to pressure areas. That was fine, because clothes would have been uncomfortable. I was always a naked sleeper anyway. Everything happened on my bed in the ICU. Eating, personal hygiene, seeing people . . . everything.

After a couple of days, I had the chance to shower. This was a big deal, because I'm one of those people who like to shower at least twice a day. I can't tolerate not showering. Oh, and here's another big scandalous secret about me while we're at it – not only do I sleep naked, but I shower naked.

The nurse got me into a shower on a bed that had blue rubber surroundings and base. I was taken into the bathroom then literally hosed down. I got a chance to shave, too. Well, to be shaved, anyway. It was nice. I felt clean again. Until that point, I didn't realise how dirty I was. There was still blood all over me. I saw it dissolving in the water. The water that swirled towards the drain looked as if a painter was washing red paint from their palette.

I wasn't allowed to eat. It wasn't safe. With the way the injury affected my body, I could choke. All I was allowed was jelly. At one point, the hospital ran out of flavoured jelly. Only thickened water was left. How does that taste, you might wonder? It tastes exactly as it sounds. Gross.

Truss came to visit me one day. He looked tired. 'Beth just had a baby. Her name is Annabelle,' he said. Beth was his wife. I cried. It was a mixture of emotions; I was happy for him, but I also knew that I was missing an important moment in my friend's life. And, I wondered if I would ever experience what Truss was feeling right then.

During that time, one important reflection kept me going.

Up till that point in my life, I did everything I could. I had really lived. I took that spur-of-the-moment trip to Japan. I asked that pretty blonde girl out in high school. I drove the fast car. I did a lot. No experience was unventured. There were enough memories to know that I had lived life to the fullest so far.

Carpe diem, baby.

I can't remember where, but I came across an interesting idea once. Say that you're 30 years old now. The average global life expectancy according to the United Nations in 2019 was 72.6 years. That means, in 2019's terms, you could potentially expect to live another 42.6 years if things went well. That sounds like a lot, but what about if it became 42 summers? How many of those summers could you guarantee living life to the fullest? Better yet, what if you told the teenage you that there were only a couple of summers left until school finished and life changed course forever? How many summers do you have with your college friends? How many summers might you have before the baby comes? How many summers do you have with your children before they leave home? Put into that context, the number starts to look precious. There's no time to waste.

I've learned that in life, tomorrow doesn't matter. Today matters. Now matters. There's no guarantee about what tomorrow will bring. There's not even a guarantee that it'll come at all. That's why it is important to seize the day. Today. Now. Up to that point in the ICU, I was glad that I had seized every day, every moment and every opportunity.

Carpe diem.

I was unstable for several days in the ICU. Every now and again, the alarms went off. The team rushed in and worked on resuscitating me. Often, it was simple things like sucking out mucus from my lungs. This was a hideously unpleasant experience. Essentially, someone ran a tube through my nose into my throat while I was awake. They sucked out any material that was inside.

Lungs are unstable in the early phases of a spinal cord injury. They fill up with gunk. Pneumonia can set in and it can then be difficult to shift. The physiotherapist came into my cubicle regularly to do chest therapy for this reason. Sometimes, they beat my chest and made me cough. Other times, they brought in a machine that did the same job. It thumped my chest until everything became loose inside. I needed it, but I hated it.

Eventually, my heart and lungs stabilised. I was ready to try and sit up.

Normally, blood redistributes in the body reasonably efficiently when you stand up. The muscles in the legs pump the blood back up to the heart, which can then pump it further to the top end – most importantly, to the brain.

The autonomic nervous system also springs into action. It stimulates the heart and blood vessels to redistribute blood to vital organs. The spinal cord is a crucial driver of all of these processes. In a spinal cord injury, these systems are broken. So, learning to be upright is a long and arduous process.

First, I sat in a big chair that could be turned flat quickly. That way, if I started to feel faint, someone could lay me flat so the blood flowed into my brain again. I remember trying to sit over and over again, but the world often greyed out as the blood pooled in the lower half of my body. Often, I was actually happy to tap out of reality for a little while.

Then, I tried a tilt table. This is a table where you lie down initially and a therapist starts to gently tilt you upright. I usually fainted. But, over about a month, my body and brain became used to being upright. I started being able to sit up more. I stopped fainting.

My lungs were also getting better. I didn't feel out of breath all the time, and I started speaking longer sentences without stopping to breathe. The flow of oxygen through the tube to my nose was gradually reduced.

Finally, they let me eat. To this day, I hold a grudge against speech pathologists. You people didn't let me eat for the longest time. I will forever remember this affront.

My friend Aimee was around when I got the clearance to eat. Aimee was a redhead. She was petite, freckled and happy. We were in medical school together. I spent a lot of time teasing her about anything and everything back in the day, but we were as thick as thieves.

'What do you want to eat?' she asked.

'Get me a steak.'

Aimee went to the pub across the road and got me a steak. It was one of the best steaks I've ever had.

Even though I was locked up in the ICU, my life outside needed some organisation. Everything was still there, suspended in uncertainty after my injury. There was medical school. My apartment. The destroyed remnants of my car. Much of this was taken on by my good friend Ben Gerhardy, now a lung specialist. Ben and I met in medical school. When the accident happened, he sprang into action to do what he could. He went to my car to fish out anything that remained. He made arrangements for my apartment. He liaised with whoever needed to be liaised with.

Today, he likes to joke that I was 'just a head' in the ICU. He uses this to marvel at how far I've come. He's right. I was really just a head back then. As a doctor himself, Ben knows what a precarious situation I was in.

Doctors often find particular things exciting. Without those things, they lose interest. For example, surgeons need things to cut. Emergency physicians need things to resuscitate. Radiologists need stimulating things to look at. Intensive care specialists need very sick people to keep alive. I was slowly becoming less sick. So gradually, the ICU doctors lost interest in me in the best ways.

I was moved down to the orthopaedic surgery ward. The spine can be dealt with by orthopaedic surgeons or neurosurgeons. I happened to be under the care of orthopaedic surgeons. Their ward was a completely different environment. In the ICU, I was in one room with one dedicated nurse. Here, I shared a bay, as well as the nursing staff, with three other people. There was one window.

I was looking out the window one day. The weather was gloomy. I remember the very moment when I thought, *When will I ever see the outside world again?* I had no idea when, or even if, this would happen. I was always restless in my life, wanting to physically move around a lot. I never even liked sleeping in the same place every day. I liked being outside as much as possible. Suddenly, I was confined to the insides of a hospital. Even if I wanted to escape, I couldn't. I was stuck there. It was the most desolate feeling.

The three other patients in my room also had spinal cord injuries. One was a young guy who had dived into a shallow pool on Australia Day. He had an injury similar to mine, but less severe. After being initially paralysed, he slowly started to move his limbs again. One night, I enviously watched him use a back scratcher to scratch his back. That little bastard. I was so itchy. I wished that I could scratch myself like he was. Simple things.

I don't remember the second patient, but I do remember the third. He was a pleasant middle-aged man. I liked him. He was flown in from somewhere far away. One morning, this man had been riding a bike to work. The front wheel of the bike hit a ditch. He was thrown off the bike and broke his spine. He was paralysed from the neck down.

His wife and daughter visited every day. In the mornings, his wife always said hello to me. She dropped fresh towels at the foot of my bed, and her thoughtfulness put a smile on my face. Our families shared the difficult journey together. We talked. We debriefed. We shared information. We shed tears.

One afternoon, we were lying in bed after finishing therapy. Therapy involved learning the basics about how to physically function while having a spinal cord injury: things like learning to use what mobility remained in my arms to do tasks and drive a wheelchair. That day, I was talking to some friends who were visiting when the alarms went off without warning. People rushed to the middle-aged man's bedside and drew the curtains. For about fifteen minutes, there was a lot of commotion. Shapes moved behind the curtains as personnel bustled about with machines and trolleys. My friends tried to distract me because I think they understood the scared look on my face. I knew what was happening. He had a cardiac arrest. The team was trying to resuscitate him, unsuccessfully.

When the curtains eventually opened again, he wasn't there anymore. That was it. The end of this man – a loved husband and father. We spoke that morning, but now he was gone forever. Life extinguished.

The emotional onslaught of the damned journey was unrelenting. For so many reasons like that, a spinal cord injury isn't an easy thing. This is especially so in the early stages, when one is trying to come to terms with what happened. In the book and movie *Me Before You*, the main character seeks euthanasia after having a spinal cord injury. This story isn't far from reality for some. In 2008, for example, a young British rugby player obtained assisted dying in Switzerland after suffering a spinal cord injury. Over the years, I've talked to people with paralysis wanting the same thing. While the statistics are not completely clear, the rate of suicide is said to be far higher in people with spinal cord injuries than those without. Although I've never thought about ending my life, I can understand why people entertain the thought. It's just not an easy road.

As hard as it was, I decided to keep going.

An academic from the medical school, Eleanor Milligan, got me access to the hospital library. She encouraged me to stay in touch with medicine and tried to find medical projects for me to do from the hospital. Eleanor and I bonded because she looked after the legal aspects of medical studies. Coming from law, I could relate to her. She was a strong, confident Scottish woman with red hair. A leader. Eleanor always supported me, before and after the accident. But I didn't take easily to her encouragement then.

I was wheeled into the library a couple of times but found it too confronting. Every time I looked at a medical book, memories came rushing back. The evenings at the university with friends, the long days bouncing exam questions off Dan, and everything around it. The pain from thinking about all that was visceral; I was now a world away, paralysed.

My days were peppered with interesting moments. For example, have you ever had someone say something completely thoughtless despite the best of intentions? One day, a friend was trying to distract me. She started telling me the story about a knee injury she just sustained. She was scheduled for surgery. 'I won't be able to walk for weeks,' she lamented. For her, it was the end of the world.

I just nodded, my forehead screwed up in concern but my mind laughing at the irony.

It was around this time that my ex-girlfriend Yaris started visiting again. She was beautiful. I often looked with awe at her slim frame and brown hair. She used to do it up in all sorts of magical ways, but it looked best when it was just a messy ball on her head. Just as always, Yaris was smart, kind and thoughtful.

Knowing that I had coeliac disease, she cooked gluten-free goodies for me. The first thing she brought me was a cake. I demolished it. By this point, I had lost about 20 kg. Weighing up again wasn't the worst thing. Yaris visited more and more. We talked a lot. She helped my mum with bits and pieces and started to come every day.

A couple of weeks into my stay in the orthopaedics ward, it was decided that I needed a second operation to fix my spine. It was still unstable. Yaris came to hang out with me on the day of the surgery. I fell asleep, went into the operating theatre, then came out without incident. This time, the back of my neck was opened up to attach a plate. Afterwards, I had another drain coming out of me. It was draining blood from the operation site.

When I opened my eyes, Yaris was there. The first thing that came to my mind was, 'You should be my girlfriend again.' It turns out that I unknowingly verbalised that thought. She said yes, and we were together again.

Dating from a hospital bed takes a lot of love. It wasn't like I could court her properly. I was a dishevelled naked guy in a gown with my ass out, learning how to master basic bodily functions again. I shared a room with three other people. The nicest place we could go out to was the hospital garden. But, Yaris was a woman with a can-do attitude.

She made me little picnics. We had candlelit dinners together. Yaris made it as romantic as she could. I remember when she made me risotto. Her mushroom risotto was spectacular. You know, risotto is an expression of love. It has to be carefully and gently stirred, sometimes over hours. The ingredients have to be just right. You make a good risotto for someone that you really love. Yaris made me risotto. She did all that while juggling medical school, exams and a job as a nurse.

Before she became a medical student, Yaris was a nurse. She had a way with people, as great nurses do. It wasn't hard for her to put people at ease. She was a natural at the whole thing.

We made the best of our circumstances. As I slowly learned how to use a wheelchair, Yaris sat on my lap while I rolled around the hospital. We kissed all the time. At night, she lay by my side until it was too late for visitors to stay. The little hospital bed could barely fit us both. I didn't care. I just wanted to hold her. Train's song 'Soul Sister' came out around then. It couldn't have been more perfect for what I thought of Yaris.

I was now in a slow tedious part of a hospital stay for a spinal cord injury. I was medically stable. There were no critical problems from my injuries. I was waiting to be transferred to the spinal injuries unit. For all of Queensland, there's only one unit specialised in the care of spinal cord injury. Patients from all around the huge state are transferred there for rehabilitation. Often, the stay lasts many months while people learn to live with their injury.

With the limited number of beds in the unit, there was normally a backlog of patients waiting to come in. Sometimes, people wait for months. Once you got a bed, then specialised rehabilitation began. One day, I was suddenly given the nod and taken down to the unit.

Despite the rush to get there, the spinal injuries unit was depressing. It was a building from the seventies or eighties and hadn't been painted in years. The inside was dark and old. One bay held four people, and while you got a bit more space than on the other wards, it was still snug. A tiny old TV hung from the ceiling. It had to be rented for a fee. The curtains were probably as old as the universe itself, and contained even more dust. The bathroom was shared with three other people. Sometimes, it was more. I felt like I entered a building that time had forgotten.

I used to get up as early as possible to get into the bathroom with the nurse. Usually, that was at about 4.30 am. The reason was that the bathrooms often weren't cleaned between patients. It wasn't unusual to find faeces everywhere. It was filthy. At least if I made it to the bathroom first thing in the morning, it was clean.

I often wondered why the spinal injuries unit was like this. People went through the hardest time of their life there. The reality is, there was probably no political will to fund its refurbishment. Even though it's one of the few places that patients will spend months and months in, the relatively low number of patients compared to other units is less likely to give anyone concern about neglect affecting votes. There's also a big power differential between the patients and the system. The patients are at the mercy of the system for such a long time, especially because there's no other service that can look after them in their time of need. It was doubtful that anyone will take a patient's feedback on meaningfully.

My three roommates were interesting. One was a young guy who was similar to me in age. The second was an Indigenous Australian from far away rural Queensland.

The third person had a host of psychiatric issues. It was a constant battle between the psychiatry unit and the spinal injuries unit as to who would take this person into their care. He was volatile and quick to anger. Many nights, I woke up to chaos. Urine was thrown at me. He threatened to kill us. Sometimes, he just stared at me for hours, his face blank. It was like there was nothing inside except hate. My one solace was that even though the distance between us was short, I knew that he couldn't get to me without support.

The place was never short of unusual experiences. One night, an intoxicated patient came into my room. He started touching my leg. 'I'm so lonely,' he said. I couldn't call out for help because no one was nearby. I just talked to him until eventually he got bored and left. These kinds of experiences weren't uncommon as a patient.

When I was once a patient in one of several hospitals for a bit of time later after the spinal cord injury, there was a notorious nurse. He was known to take young less-mobile male patients into their beds to 'clean the little man'. It didn't matter whether it was day or night. If he saw you, there was a good chance that the little man was going to get cleaned – whether he needed it or not. At night, though, there was no choice. The little man invariably got a clean. It happened to me more than once. I'm going to give this man the benefit of the doubt by thinking that he had a particular interest in male genital hygiene. But some have suggested that this was sexual abuse.

When I thought of writing about this, I messaged a friend who had also been a patient in that same hospital. He shared experiencing similar stories, then concluded by saying, 'See, places like that are so messed up you don't even know what's abuse and what's not.'

This sadly is unsurprising. According to the Australian Institute of Health and Welfare, as of 2016, about 43 per cent of adults with a disability and 50 per cent of adults with a severe disability experienced sexual harassment. In comparison, 37 per cent of adults without a disability experienced sexual harassment. People with disability are at high risk of sexual abuse both within and outside institutional settings.

Those sobering statistics aside, the little man was a big topic sometimes. One day, I was doing physiotherapy. I was in a standing frame with the therapist in front of me. Completely unintentionally, the little man stood to attention for the first time since the accident. I had no control of it, but the autonomic nervous system had sprung into action, activating the little man. It was clear for everyone to see through my shorts, now a tent.

'I'm so sorry, it's not you,' I said. 'Not that you're not attractive, but it just happened,' I added to the train wreck.

'Don't worry, this happens all the time,' the therapist gently replied.

It was like being in high school again.

News of the little man spread like wildfire that day. I got

text messages saying things like, *I just heard. Congratulations.* Visitors came that evening bearing gifts, saying, 'We heard the great news today.' A community gathered around the little man, celebrating his resurrection.

As nights in the unit were not peaceful, I became hyper-vigilant. The smallest sound woke me up. Mum and Yaris hunted down some construction worker earmuffs to drown out any noise. I also wore an eye cover.

Rehabilitation was slow. We had one to two hours of physiotherapy per day. Added to that was one to two hours of occupational therapy, focusing mainly on hand function. The rest of the time was spent hovering aimlessly around the spinal injuries unit. Sometimes, there were other things to attend to like arranging a new wheelchair.

Every day, we trudged on. Mum lived about an hour away in 8 Mile. She cooked me food in the morning then drove straight over in time for when I was getting up. She stayed with me all day then drove home at night. She was doing this every single day. Luckily, my grandma flew in from Sri Lanka around then to keep Mum company. At least she had moral support and someone to share the drive with. Like Mum, Grandma was strong. Apparently, Grandma said to my crying mum once, 'Why are you crying? You have no time to cry. You need to get moving and get that boy sorted.' After that, Mum didn't cry.

Eventually, Mum's employer said that a choice had to be made. Mum had to keep working or she would lose her job.

She needed her job, but she also wanted to look after me. In spite of the ultimatum, Mum somehow continued to juggle both work and me. It was difficult for her.

I hated being inside the spinal injuries unit. Luckily, I was able to go outside in a wheelchair by this point so I usually went out to the garden with Mum. I spent most of the day out there. I never knew that I could get a tan, but being in the sun constantly made me very dark. On top of just being away from the unit, I just liked being in the sun. With a spinal cord injury, the ability for the skin to control body temperature is lost. That means you become somewhat cold-blooded, like a lizard. Cold environments are the worst. Warm environments are bliss. The simple things made the biggest difference.

It sometimes doesn't take much to make a patient happy. To give someone dignity. For them to feel like they matter. The little things count the most: a clean bathroom, a warm blanket. I often think of this at work in the emergency department.

One night, I was working with a nurse who was an old battleaxe. She took no prisoners. A patient with some psychiatric problems came in. He was agitated. He already had some rib fractures from an altercation with security guards elsewhere. When the patient came into the cubicle, things were escalating. The intern felt that it was beyond their scope. They came to get me for help, as I was the most senior person around.

When the patient and I spoke, he calmed down. He said that no one had listened to him. He knew that no one could help him with the psychiatric problems, but he was hungry and just wanted a sandwich. If he got a sandwich, he would leave peacefully.

At this point, Nurse Battleaxe walked in. She said that there was no way the patient would be getting a sandwich.

'I'm just going to go kill myself,' the patient said.

'Good. Do us all a favour,' retorted Battleaxe.

Things escalated again. Security were brought in. It became ugly – unnecessarily so.

The solution was so simple. A terrible two-dollar hospital sandwich in return for a happy patient with no violence. Sadly, attitudes – and perhaps egos – got in the way.

Another night, I was the doctor for a young patient whose metastatic cancer had suddenly become significantly worse. After many years of being stable, the prognosis was grim. This was unexpected to them and their partner. The partner buried their head in their hands. Both began to cry. I couldn't hold back my tears. We cried together silently.

I wonder if some of our patients realise that we will always remember them. Just like this patient, my soul is burned with the memories of so many people who I've connected with even just for a few hours.

We talked about what they needed. The patient just wanted to be out of pain. Still, we needed to do another scan to figure out some other potentially treatable issues.

I stepped away from the patient to organise the scan. In that time, another Battleaxe had walked into the cubicle. An issue unnecessarily started to brew. The Battleaxe wanted the patient's partner out. Those were the rules during COVID times, apparently. The partner didn't want to leave. We all knew that this was potentially the beginning of a terminal event. They wanted to be together.

After an argument with the Battleaxe, we finally agreed that the partner would stay. I wondered, when do we lose our hearts? I know that there are rules. Yet, we need to keep our humanity intact while navigating those rules. Ironically, our hospital's motto is 'We Care Always'.

I debriefed about this event with one of my bosses. She said that maybe the Battleaxe was dealing with other pressures. Maybe the department was short on beds. Maybe they had some personal issues. I get that. But, I don't think that it's any excuse to treat a patient facing a terminal event – the end of their life – with less love. This is the end of the road for them. The hospital will always keep rolling.

Most of us just want to be heard. I just wanted some simple comforts like a clean bathroom in the place where I was to spend many months. I experienced this lack of dignity all the time when I was in the unit. No, the room couldn't be changed so I could be away from the guy throwing urine at me. I was a young guy and should be equipped to handle it, they implied.

My therapy was slow, but I was learning to use the wheelchair better. I was learning to do some things with my hands, even though my fingers weren't working. I learned to transfer into a car. Yaris was eager to take me for a drive. We figured out how to jump into her little black car. She packed a cheese board. We drove up into the mountains nearby and had a picnic on the dashboard. Those little things made a huge difference. They connected me to the world outside.

Until we figured out how to get in the car, I was using accessible taxis to do short trips in the vicinity of the hospital. This wasn't cheap, though. A short trip could easily amount to fifty dollars. A long trip could cost hundreds. The taxi drivers rarely followed all the safety requirements; there wasn't much care taken when tying the wheelchair into the cab. We had several close calls and I nearly fell on many occasions.

Driving in the rain initially brought back memories of the accident. I felt on edge as my body tuned into hard-wired responses of fear and panic. But as I did it more and more, the feelings melted away. These days, I love driving in the rain.

While I was in the spinal injuries unit, one of my law school buddies, Greg, got married. Greg asked me to be his groomsman. 'I don't care if you come in a hospital bed, but I want you by my side,' he said. On the morning of the wedding, I dressed in a suit for the first time since the accident. To make things interesting, Greg was getting married on an island. After we drove out to a jetty, Mum and Grandma lowered me into a tiny boat with Yaris. The shaky boat took us to the island.

I was somehow manoeuvred onto the beach where the ceremony happened. It was beautiful. Afterwards, Yaris and I watched people dance at the reception. There were many couples in love. They twirled. They hugged, bathed by the soft fairy lights. We sat by the side of it all, knowing that we couldn't be a part of that dance in that way. In one moment, I looked at Yaris's eyes and saw pain. I knew why.

'I get what you're thinking,' I said.

'It's okay. I'll get over it. I just need some time.'

No more words needed to be said.

As the months passed, I became secure in my new environment at the unit. My entire sense of self had changed. The daily routine and long time in the hospital created a feeling of security. I didn't want to leave. I was institutionalised. Mum started encouraging me to come home on weekends, as was allowed by the hospital. I was terrified at first. I didn't want to face the world. I didn't feel safe.

Eventually, Mum coaxed me into the family home on a Friday night. Despite my fears, it felt great. I was in my own bed. I felt normal. I gradually started spending more and more days at home. After a while, I was spending more time at home than at the hospital. I slept at home then went back to the hospital for therapy during the day. I was still technically a patient there with an allocated bed, but I was only there part-time.

One morning, I woke up at home. I felt strange. I was sweating profusely, and the sweat wouldn't stop. It was a winter's day, which made the sweat even more unusual. I started feeling worse and worse. My skin felt uncomfortable and my chest was tight. By the time we got to the hospital, I was feeling terrible. The nurses scanned my bladder to find that it was retaining urine. I deteriorated more. My vital signs became unstable.

This phenomenon is called autonomic dysreflexia. In a high-level spinal cord injury, any painful stimulus below the level of the injury causes the body to go haywire. This is because pain causes adrenaline to stream out uncontrollably. Normally, the brain will dampen down that adrenaline. But in a spinal cord injury, the brain can't send that signal down, so the body just keeps releasing adrenaline. The blood pressure goes through the roof. The heart beats slower in response. If it's not treated promptly, it can lead to death. It's a medical emergency. This is what was happening to me.

Severe autonomic dysreflexia is terrifying. Many patients who I've seen with the complication are acutely scared that they'll die. When I've had it, I, too, felt like I was on the verge of death. The feeling comes over you like a slow black fog filling you up inside. Then, you start to sweat. The worse it gets, the more you sweat. My sheets have been soaked with it at times. As the blood pressure rises, a headache forms. Your chest becomes tight. You can feel your heart pounding. You know that if something isn't done, bad things will happen – the worst being something like a bleed in the brain. That happened to someone I met in the spinal injuries unit. They died in their sleep when it hit, only in their twenties.

The staff were desperate to try to get an intravenous line into me to give me some drugs. But everything was shut down. A nurse made a last-ditch effort and successfully put a line in my foot. They were able to stabilise me through that line with fluids and medications.

This episode was a setback. It was a reminder that any sense of physiological stability I had was still brittle. But once I recovered, I persevered with easing out of hospital bit by bit. I kept going back to the house. I slept there more. Eventually, my hospital bed was given to another patient, one who was earlier in their journey than I was. I was discharged after around seven or eight months in that place.

I was back in the real world.

4

HEALING THE SOUL

We will only understand the miracle of life fully when
we allow the unexpected to happen.

Paulo Coelho

I REMEMBER LYING in bed at home, back at my parents'
place in 8 Mile, not long after being discharged from the
hospital. It was a sunny day. I saw trees outside. I was star-
fished lengthwise on the bed with my laptop on my chest.
Out of the blue, a realisation hit me. *I can't move. Even if
I try, I can't get up out of the bed. I can't sit up. I'm stuck in
this position. I can't reach the beauty of nature outside by my
own power. And, I don't know when that will change.* It was a
horrifying thought. Even though the thought wasn't like a
sledgehammer constantly banging away like when I was in
the ICU, it still surfaced occasionally in those days.

I was watching the movie *Invictus* on the laptop. Every
time I see it now, I think of that day on the bed. It's amazing

how something like a song or movie can anchor a memory so vividly in the soul. *Invictus* also has a special meaning for me. When I was in the hospital, a friend hung up the poem of the same name, which is recited in the movie, by my bed. It goes like this.

> Out of the night that covers me
> Black as the pit from pole to pole,
> I thank whatever gods may be
> For my unconquerable soul.
> In the fell clutch of circumstance,
> I have not winced nor cried aloud.
> Under the bludgeonings of chance
> My head is bloody, but unbowed.
> Beyond this place of wrath and tears
> Looms but the Horror of the shade,
> And yet the menace of the years
> Finds, and shall find, me unafraid.
> It matters not how strait the gate,
> How charged with punishments the scroll,
> I am the master of my fate:
> I am the captain of my soul.

The story is that the author of the poem, William Ernest Henley, lost a leg due to complications from tuberculosis. Later, he nearly lost the other leg, but the famous surgeon Joseph Lister was able to save it. While recovering from this second episode, Henley wrote the poem in the hospital. The word 'Invictus' means 'invincible' or 'undefeated' in Latin. The poem also forms a foundation for the Invictus Games, which celebrate the spirit of injured servicepeople.

The words in the poem have had a profound effect on me. They remind me that regardless of what happens, I am the captain of my soul – and that simple acts of kindness can make a big difference in a person's life. It was such a simple gesture for my friend to pin up a poem printed on an A4 sheet of paper by my hospital bed. Not only did it touch my heart, but I'm writing about it years later in a book. We all have the opportunity to leave an imprint like that on another person. Every day. While our presence in each other's lives can be fleeting, those impressions can last a lot longer – much like my relationship with Yaris.

Yaris and I were happily together by then. She stayed with me at night, then went to the hospital to be a medical student in the morning. She woke up in the wee hours of the morning, at around 4 am, to get to the hospital in time. I watched her get ready in my room, putting her hair in that cute bun. Then, she was away. After she left, I slept a bit more. We had no help except my grandma. Mum came back from work during her lunch break to help me up. I waited for her again to go to physiotherapy in the afternoon. The clinic was an hour away. Mum, Grandma and I joked in the car during the long drive. I always dreaded getting out of the car because of the cold weather. I shivered all the way from the car park to the clinic. Yaris often met me at the clinic after medical school. 'Come on, baby, you want to be strong for me, right?' she encouraged me, just like Mum and Grandma. Yaris sat with her laptop studying while I did therapy. We spent a couple of hours at the clinic before going home. Those were our days.

We used to have a big white cat at home. He was huge – at least 12 kilograms. His name was Alby, and he was my friend. After the accident, he wouldn't leave my side. If I was in bed, he lay at the foot of the bed. If the door was shut, he scratched at it until someone let him in. He came into the shower. When I got in the car to go somewhere, he jumped in the car. Alby must've known that I was injured. He tried to be there for me.

Mum and I talked about the next steps all the time. We eventually figured that it might be a good idea to visit Sri Lanka temporarily. After fifteen years, we could be with our relatives. They had offered to help. There would be some security for us in having more help. At the same time, we heard whispers of ayurvedic medicine doing wonders for people with spinal cord injuries. When there was nothing to lose and nothing left to try, we decided to go to Sri Lanka.

A spinal cord injury is a great teacher of many things, and one lesson is about having nothing left to lose. In medicine, we always see people trying desperate measures to cure terrible diseases. Spinal cord injury is no different. I have close friends who spent hundreds of thousands of dollars going around the world to try all kinds of treatments that promise to cure paralysis. I don't think that there is a right or wrong to that. When I was desperate, I wanted to try everything too. Even if there was a sliver of a chance that it might work, my family was willing to give it a shot.

The flipside to that is that there are often people profiting from the vulnerable. People sell their homes. People use their entire insurance payout. Communities gather to collect money. We've all come across these stories. All this money sadly sometimes ends up in a questionable character's pocket. I met many questionable characters on my journey. They came out of the woodwork, especially at the start.

I once met a guy who claimed to be a neurologist in London's famous Harley Street. He was introduced to me by an actual neurologist, which gave him some credibility. The guy was apparently travelling around the world to set up a revolutionary treatment that used an implant to translate signals from the brain to the spinal cord to restore function. Funnily enough, this concept is not as outlandish today as it was then. Nonetheless, the good 'professor' wanted five hundred thousand dollars to give me the treatment. Jesse, the schoolfriend I skipped class with, was involved in this conversation at some point and even offered to sell his house to pay for it.

I quickly became suspicious of our globe-trotting professor because he didn't have even the most basic grasp of brain anatomy during our conversations. I looked deep into his website, which boasted numerous awards from various institutions. When I contacted the institutions, they'd never heard of him. Even though he claimed to have been awarded an 'Albert Schweitzer Prize for Humanitarianism in 2005', for example, the organisation confirmed that this was a lie. When I dug deeper, I found that he was wanted by the London police for stealing money from retirees in nursing homes. He was a seasoned conman. I contacted the London police, but as he was then based somewhere outside their area of jurisdiction, they couldn't do anything about him.

He wasn't the only charlatan I came across. Shamans asked for thousands of dollars to perform rituals that would surely make me walk again. Glamorous new-age churches promised that I could be healed. And if I couldn't, it was because I didn't have faith.

This goes on constantly. Vulnerable people are taken advantage of. It's a sad side of human nature. Even though I have medical training, legal training and a solid education, the desperation of a difficult situation tempted me.

Still, people need hope. Vietnamese Buddhist monk and peace activist Thích Nhất Hạnh said, 'Hope is important because it can make the present moment less difficult to bear. If we believe that tomorrow will be better, we can bear a hardship today.'

As a junior doctor, I once cared for a very young patient with metastatic cancer. They had no idea it was growing inside them until they turned up in our emergency department, suddenly ill. By then, it was everywhere. I went to say hello months later while they were getting chemotherapy in the hospital. The whole family was with the patient. When I asked how they were, the father of this patient told me, 'Don't worry. I have a secret weapon.' He pointed up, signifying God. They would pray. God will save them, the patient's dad said. I hoped with all my heart that something would come through for them. Sadly, the patient passed away.

In medicine, we're sometimes quick to take away hope from people. But I know that hope gave the entire family strength when they needed it most.

But even outside medicine, we're quick to take away hope. The basketball coach who tells the teenager that they will never make the big league. The friends who tell the actress that she will never make it to Hollywood. The teacher who tells the student that they are doomed to fail. The investor who tells the entrepreneur that their idea is ridiculous. How many times have you heard the story of the adult who told a child that they would never amount to anything? I know that I've been told something similar more than once.

In my first year of university way back when, I struggled with a subject. My grades were sagging. I approached a lecturer for help. He was quick to anger, saying that he didn't have time for people like me. I don't know what he meant by people 'like me', but he proceeded to suggest that I wouldn't make much of myself. There was no point, he said, in him investing any time in me. Much later, after many milestones in my life, I emailed him. I told him who I became. It was a bittersweet moment. While he couldn't remember me, he replied and apologised for his attitude of the past. We must be careful when we hand out judgements to people, especially when there's a power differential.

Anyway, who are we to take away people's hope for a better tomorrow? Who are we to take away what could make the hardship of today bearable for someone?

Mum, Grandma and I decided to chase hope and security, with hope making our hardship more bearable. We thought that we would find it back in Sri Lanka. So, we booked our tickets and packed our bags – and quickly learned about the challenges of travelling with a spinal cord injury. We needed a heap of equipment: emergency medical supplies, a wheelchair for the shower, dressings for wounds . . . the list went on. We got it all ready. Sometime in August or September 2010, we lugged everything to the airport.

Airlines can be difficult to deal with. They rarely understand the intricacies of travelling with a wheelchair. Often, equipment is damaged in transit. More than once, I've landed at an airport to find a destroyed wheelchair. Airlines usually respond by saying, 'Just hire one'. They don't realise that a wheelchair is specifically prescribed to ensure that its user doesn't develop sometimes life-threatening wounds or encounter other safety issues. If you search online, there are stories of wheelchair users dying from complications of such neglect during air travel. Standard wheelchairs also cost tens of thousands of dollars. An electric wheelchair can set you back hundreds of thousands of dollars.

Mum and Grandma managed to get me into an aeroplane seat with some help. First we travelled from Brisbane to Singapore. There we tried to rush from one gate to another. Mum and Grandma both had many bags. They were trying to push me in the wheelchair at the same time, and Grandma fell. Fortunately, she didn't hurt herself, and we managed to get to the next gate in time. We were finally on a plane to Sri Lanka.

When we landed in Colombo, my uncle picked us up in a rental car. It was a small Toyota sedan, commonplace in Sri Lanka. It was so long since I had been there – it felt like a lifetime. Plus, Sri Lanka had changed. It was like a new world for me. We drove through the bustling streets lined with food stalls. Even in the late hours of the night, there was plenty of activity. Decrepit old buses with people hanging out of them filled the streets. The occasional Buddhist monk walked by, draped in their orange robes. The air was thick with all sorts of exotic smells, like the rich smoke from deep-fried street food mixing with exhaust fumes from the overpacked vehicles. It was a sensory buffet. Colombo was hot and humid. I loved it. I didn't have to be scared of being cold anymore.

We stayed in a hotel, because we needed somewhere reliably accessible. Long-lost relatives flocked to visit us. These were people who I hadn't seen for 15 years. I had no strong memories of anyone. While some were genuinely happy to see us, I felt uneasy about others. Something just didn't seem right. There was a note of disingenuity behind their eyes.

Days started to tick by, and Mum and I settled in. Grandma stayed with us. After paying the routine visits for a few days, some relatives started asking for money. These were the ones I felt uneasy about. We were running on credit cards ourselves by that point, but we naïvely helped out a few, not knowing that this would prompt a never-ending stream of requests. Because we were from Australia, we were perceived to be rich by default.

Around this time, I had some difficult thoughts about Yaris. We were still talking by phone, but things became strained. It wasn't her but me.

The experience at Greg's wedding stewed in my mind for a long time. I wanted Yaris to have a normal life. Life with me wasn't normal. It wasn't fair to drag her into it. Everything with a spinal cord injury is different. We couldn't hold hands and walk on the beach. We couldn't dance together. Intimacy was different. She didn't care, but I cared. My attitude now is very different, but that's how I felt then. So, I let her go.

Today, I know that she has a normal life with a husband and many children. To my knowledge, she's happy. I have no feelings for her now. I don't think about her anymore, but we shared something unique together for a brief time. For that, I'm grateful.

After a few weeks, still holed up in the hotel in Sri Lanka, Mum's employer asked her to come back to work. If she didn't, she would have to quit. At the same time, several people in our lives were even encouraging Mum to put me in a Sri Lankan nursing home. I still have a copy of one email. *He will be fine in a nursing home. You need to keep your job*, it said to Mum. She was in a difficult position.

We decided that Mum would go back to Australia to work until we figured out a plan, whatever that was going to be. I couldn't go back with her because we had no support at home then. I was to stay with our relatives in Sri Lanka. We hired a nurse to come in and help me once a day. The relatives promised to hang out with me in an apartment that we rented. My grandma stayed as well.

Mum cried on the way to the airport. She promised me that she would be back. I said that it was okay, that we'd get through it. But, I hated to see her go.

I was staying in an apartment that was about thirty years old, and it was starting to show its age. The walls were peeling in some places, the carpet was stained, and some of the bath-room tiles were cracked. The colours were dark and the lights dim. Having said that, the apartment was in a brilliant loca-tion, right in the middle of Colombo. It faced the sea. Every day, I watched the sun go down over the Indian Ocean.

I spent most of my time lying in bed staring out at the ocean. A few weeks went by. There wasn't any help for me to get around, because the nurse was only coming for a very limited time. Some relatives were still around, more to take money than to help. I lay there thinking about life. I still had no idea what to do next.

One night, the relatives came to my room. They knew that the money supply was drying up. They said that they could no longer help me, and just like that, they left. They took my wallet, my bank card, and what little cash I had. I was alone. Later, we found out that one of them had even been lying about the cost of groceries for me. He'd been ripping us off for weeks. On the other side of the world, Mum was terribly distressed at the situation.

Mum and I decided to keep going as things were. The nurse was still coming. They came in the evening, stayed through the night, then left in the morning.

Throughout the day, I often struggled with the cold. Even though Colombo was warm, the sun didn't shine into my room until late afternoon. The air conditioning had no heating capability because it just wasn't required in Colombo, and even if it had, I couldn't have reached it.

Sometimes, I covered my face with a pillow. I could still feel warmth on my face, so a pillow reduced the sensation of being cold. There was a period of weeks where I was constantly sweating and shivering. I had no other symptoms at all. In retrospect, I was probably ill with some kind of infection. Luckily, it went away after some time.

I didn't eat through the day. There was no one to help me with food. Fortunately, I was rarely hungry.

My laptop became my best friend. It connected me to the world and kept me entertained. A lot of friends stopped contacting me and replying to my emails. They stopped picking up my calls. But Dean, Jesse, Truss, Ben and Dan made an effort to regularly keep in touch. Their phone calls meant a lot. Jesse encouraged me to think about the future. 'Imagine when you come back!' he always said excitedly. 'Imagine when you get back to medical school.' He was forever the optimist, one that I needed. I emailed Mum all the time.

I had movies, books and the internet too. I read a lot. The story of *The Count of Monte Cristo* struck a particular chord with me. If you haven't read it, it's a great story. Considered a classic novel, it's about a man who was betrayed by people close to him. He ended up in a terrible island prison called Château d'If. He eventually escaped from the prison with the help of a monk. The monk, who died, pointed him to a hidden treasure beforehand. The man retrieved the treasure, became the Count of Monte Cristo, then took revenge on the people who betrayed him. I wasn't so much interested in revenge, but coming back better than ever.

In his book *Ego is the Enemy*, Ryan Holiday writes about the concept of 'alive time' and 'dead time'. Dead time is where something difficult happens to you, but you wait passively for it to pass. You lament that the situation sucks. You wallow. You despair. Time goes by without anything happening. Alive time is instead using that time to do something positive. You learn. You grow. You make the best out of a bad situation. Holiday talks about Malcolm X's time in prison to illustrate the point. Apparently, Malcolm X described prison as the place where he felt most free. In prison, Malcolm X read about a range of topics like religion and sociology. It was his university. It's where he grew to become the person we know. If he didn't do that, allowing time to just pass in prison, we would have lost that historical figure.

I tried to transform my dead time in Sri Lanka into alive time. And really, it became a whole other period of education.

I read books about philosophy, business, art, religion, politics and anything about people. I read about values. I read about perseverance. I read about strength. I reflected on my flaws. I realised that there was a lot of character-building that I needed to do. I settled on a bunch of non-negotiable values I wanted to stick with. These were things like integrity, loyalty and perseverance. Loyalty, because I felt betrayed and abandoned by many when the injury happened. Perseverance, because I felt that's what I needed the most to get through this. Integrity, because I learned that it is one of the fundamental building blocks of being a good human being. I wrote these down. I read about them every day. I wanted to become better.

It's important to understand our principles, to explicitly know them. It's actually what religion is about to a certain extent. Think about the Ten Commandments. Ten principles to live by. Even Buddhism has five precepts. It's a good thing to know our principles, but it's another thing to uphold them every day. The world has a way of testing our resolve frequently. That's when our principles matter the most.

Let me give you an example I came across years later. There was a man who helped me a great deal. In fact, I could argue that I wouldn't be here sharing this story with you if it weren't for him. He was an impressive man with a career behind him that took him to stratospheric heights. When he reached the sky, I noticed hubris creeping in. Our conversations were tinged with shades of overconfidence and entitlement. Eventually, he cheated on his wife. He began to lie. He stole. Then, he asked me to lie for him as well. He asked me to compromise myself more than once, for example by providing dodgy references or to lie to others to gain him an advantage. The requests became frequent. I thought long and hard. How do I turn away someone who has done so much for me? How do I balance loyalty with integrity? I still don't have the right answer. In the end, I told him that although I owed him much, I couldn't compromise my integrity for him. And with that note, our relationship disintegrated.

While I was using my alive time to grow in Sri Lanka, my situation wasn't getting any better. Then, help came in an unexpected way.

One day, the building manager for my apartment came to my place. She noticed that I was lying in a filthy state, alone.

The apartment was a mess. I had no food. She quickly told the owner of the apartment. To my surprise, the owner was someone from Brisbane, back home in Australia. I'll call him Jack. He was the head of a large company, and a genius who performed all sorts of financial wizardry.

Jack happened to be in Sri Lanka at the time, and he came to investigate my situation. He was saddened. Jack told me that I could have the apartment rent-free until my mum and I got back on our feet. He took off doors to make it more accessible. He told me to let him know whatever I needed to make life easier. Jack was a kind and generous man.

At the same time, some of our financial pressures eased. This was in part thanks to Jack. The other part was from a small insurance settlement that came through from the car accident. Mum was able to leave her job and come back to Colombo. We were reunited. I can't describe the happiness of having Mum back. It felt like home again. We started making incremental steps to regaining some sort of normalcy.

Not too long after Mum came back, Jack tragically had a sudden illness. He lost the ability to walk and use a hand too. Like me, he started using a wheelchair, which turned his world upside down.

I watched Jack go through the same experience I did. An interesting thing was how the people around him reacted. Jack was successful, wealthy in more ways than one. Some days, his house was full of sports stars, politicians and actresses.

But after the illness, and over time, these people left him. There was nothing to gain. The house became empty.

Some people betrayed him in the worst of ways. Jack once helped a young guy, put him through education at one of the most prestigious universities in the world, then developed his career into the leader of a corporate powerhouse. From my perspective, this man's entire success had stemmed from Jack's kindness. But after Jack had the illness, the guy gradually began to lose patience with him. Eventually, he was involved in removing Jack from many of his leadership positions. In the end, Jack lost a lot quickly. I wished that his kindness and generosity to me had given him some karmic protection, but it didn't.

We sometimes see this in society, don't we? The big headline of the famous person falling from grace. When someone falls, society sometimes helps them fall hard. Maybe *Schadenfreude* is more real than we think.

Buddhism teaches that everything is impermanent; everything is transient. Our lives are like that. Social status is particularly prone to the fickle fancies of the world. That's why humility is so important. How many leaders do we see ignoring the people who helped elevate them to their position? How many celebrities do we see brushing off their fans? How many bosses treat their staff terribly? Hubris is a terrible risk to take, because tomorrow you could quickly and brutally be brought back to earth. I've seen it so many times.

But, there are people who choose humility over hubris even when they have the greatest opportunity not to. A mum once reached out to me. Her child had a rare genetic disorder. As he grows, he'll need a wheelchair more and more. His mum wanted to know how she could encourage him to live a fulfilling life. I agreed to meet them. We met at a café to talk about his future. I asked the little guy what he wanted to do when he grew up. He had the very specific dream of wanting to be the CEO of one of Australia's most well-known multibillion-dollar companies. I decided to contact the then CEO about this boy's dream. The CEO wrote back to me immediately, on a Sunday evening. He offered to talk to the lad. He also arranged for the little one to explore one of their facilities. They gave him some gifts, including a T-shirt that said 'future CEO'.

This is leadership. This is humility. There's no arrogance, no hubris, just the CEO of a multibillion-dollar organisation changing the life of one child. If that CEO ever fell, we would put our arms out to catch him.

Similarly, I met an executive from another large Australian company. He was previously an executive in a different company which had fallen into trouble. He lost his job. All the people who had previously fed off his position of power stopped taking his calls. When he reached out to people to ask for help, they were too busy. He became alone. Still, this guy had guts. So, he climbed his way back to the top of the corporate ladder. Today, once again back on top, this executive cherishes the philosophy that no one is ever too busy to help another person. He always – always – opens the door to anyone who knocks, as he says.

In contrast, I have a friend from university who loves to talk about how busy he is. Every time I talk to him, I hear tales about busyness. Often, he doesn't answer when I call. He doesn't reply to text messages. He doesn't reply to emails. And when he does? You guessed it. I hear about how busy he is.

Busyness is a funny thing in our culture. It's worn like a badge of honour. But I choose not to use that word. Saying that I'm busy could give someone the message that there are more important things in my life than them, or that I have an inflated sense of self-importance. Neither of those things is true.

Moreover, the word busy takes power away from me. It means that the way I spend time is outside my control, which isn't correct. I choose what I do. If not, I'd be a slave. If you're a slave in Ancient Egypt, forced to build the pharaoh's pyramid, then you're busy. If you're a child forced to work in a sweat shop, then you're busy. Me living in a privileged country, pursuing dreams of my choice, is not busyness. It's a privilege. Therefore, I'm never busy. If the CEO of that company wasn't too busy to help a child, then I'm not busy for anyone either.

After I had the accident, many people were too busy for me. I lost plenty of friends. I had no social standing. People who I had considered close drifted away. I was sad, even a little bit bitter. I cut off the superficial aspects of my social life. I deleted my social media accounts. I started making more time for the people who were there for me. After I did that, I met more people who truly mattered.

Jack had some fascinating friends in Colombo. He introduced me to Dilith, Sarva and Varuni. I still wasn't in a state, mostly emotionally, to face the world. When they first came to visit me, I was lying naked in bed. The only thing covering me was a sheet. We still joke about that.

They spoke to me about their life. Dilith and Varuni were lawyers. While in law school, they started a small advertising business called Triad. The starting capital was just a couple of hundred dollars. They had a desk in a small office. Initially, they made simple flyers for businesses. Over time, their humble business grew into an empire. They ended up having, among other things, some of the largest media outlets in Sri Lanka as well as the oldest company in the country. The company registration number on the certificate was simply, '1'.

Sarva in particular took an interest in me. He was Dilith and Varuni's CEO. Sarva was well known in his circles for having a big heart. He and Mum plotted how to get me back into the world. At that point, it was about a year and half after the accident. I had been back in Sri Lanka for just under a year. I still wasn't ready to go out into the world. I was securely hiding away.

This isn't uncommon after something like a spinal cord injury. Many years afterwards when I was back in Australia, I got an email from a children's hospital. They had a boy with a new spinal cord injury. They asked if I could go and say hello to him. Of course, I did. Seeing the lad made me sad for him. He was so young, just a kid. He hadn't lived at all. I experienced so much life before my injury. This little guy, less than ten, had never even held a girl's hand.

What was most thought-provoking was the fact that he hadn't looked in a mirror after the injury. For over eighteen months, I, too, didn't look in a mirror. It was hard to face myself, to look at myself again. Before the accident, I was admittedly pretty vain. After the accident, my entire body changed. I always wondered, how would the world see me? I didn't even want to see myself. I think that was part of the reason I hid away in Sri Lanka for so long.

Around this time, Ben visited Sri Lanka. He came to spend some time in a general hospital as a visiting student. He chose the country so he would have the chance to see me. When Ben arrived, I didn't want him to see me in a wheelchair. He was there for several weeks, but I kept avoiding him. Thankfully, he understood why: I wasn't ready to face him.

Sarva kept prodding me to come out, and Mum joined him. I had only known Sarva for a couple of months then, but he asked me to come to work at Triad. One day, I gave in. I only gave in because Sarva was so persistent. I decided to go to his office. He prepared a desk for me and explained what they did. Their business was creating advertising for brands. I quickly found the work interesting.

Triad was a hive of creativity. At the heart of the company's ethos was the desire to remain local; to give their communication a Sri Lankan touch. Sarva got me involved in some of their projects and I started going to work more and more. It was a steep learning curve; advertising was a whole new thing for me.

For a long time, I had simply been living inside an apartment in Colombo. But very quickly after I started working, I started really living in Colombo proper. This was the start of an unexpected but happy time in my journey.

5

THE DREAM CALLING

> What man actually needs is not a tensionless state but rather the striving and struggling for some goal worthy of him.
>
> Viktor Frankl

THE EARLY 2010S was an interesting time to be in Sri Lanka. In 2009, the civil war ended. After the war, the country experienced an economic boom. In 2002, 13 per cent of Sri Lankans lived in extreme poverty: that is, having less than US$1.25 per person per day. In 2019, that number had dropped to about 4 per cent. The unemployment rate dropped after the war as well, and the value of the stock exchange boomed. Tourism increased. The excitement in the country was palpable.

In Colombo, Sri Lanka's largest city, new buildings were quickly going up everywhere. Luxury apartment buildings were becoming commonplace, although their sale price and rents were comparable to Australia and therefore out of reach for most Sri Lankans. Luxury cars, luxury goods, big brands – it was all there. Even major global artists were starting to tour the country. Having said this, general living costs were also sometimes comparable to Australia, and that was a big deal, because at the time, most Sri Lankan incomes were still a tiny fraction of what Australians earned.

The contrast in wealth was obvious at times. I knew a guy in Colombo who lived in an apartment worth at least US$1 million then. He drove a rare European sports car. One day, he bought a watch rumoured to be worth about US$2 million dollars. It was reportedly flown in and hand-delivered to him. I find this easy to believe, because even luxe watchmakers like Jaeger-LeCoultre had a presence in Colombo.

The difficulty for me was hearing this story, then driving down the street and seeing people begging for food on the roadside. Mum and I often went to certain parts of the city to distribute food to the poor. People always flocked to eat.

Streets away, there were ultra-wealthy churches and temples. The wealthy spent thousands of dollars at these places hoping for a better life, even though their situations were already comfortable, while the poor starved. Religion is a funny thing this way, I think. The fundamental principles preached in most religions are good: tolerance. Love. Peace. Giving. But then, I met the likes of one woman who went to church clutching her Michael Kors handbag and prayed for a new BMW.

'God can give you anything,' she told me. 'The poor are poor because they are sinners.'

Seriously?

I felt a sense of darkness in some of these cult-like groups, which I visited every now and again. Many were offering to make me walk again. Often, I just went out of sheer curiosity. It was a true perversion of religion, praying on people's vulnerabilities.

Trying to be a good human being is far more valuable than carrying out rituals in the hope that a greater power will yield to our selfish whims. Who really is a better Christian? The lady praying for a BMW or the one volunteering at a soup kitchen every second day?

All that aside, the Sri Lanka of those days made my work with Sarva interesting. I had the opportunity to work on projects with brands like James Packer's Crown, Shangri-La, Porsche and many iconic Sri Lankan companies. I learned the business of business.

I was fascinated by the way in which business deals were done. In law school, everything had to have a precedent. If you made a statement, it had to be backed by case law or legislation. Even when backed by both, you often have to justify it further. Current medical practice too is founded on the best available evidence, which comes from scientific research. An unfounded statement is readily questioned by a peer – frequently in public. In the absolute worst-case scenario, wrong information can lead to someone's death.

Business was a little different. In the business world, people are often trying to sell each other something. That something could be an idea, a product or even a business itself. The story of something is really important in business. Multimillion-dollar deals are sometimes made or not made based on a good story.

For example, FC Barcelona liked Lionel Messi's story so much, they signed him up in a hurry – the contract on a napkin – at the age of thirteen. He's gone on to become one of the greatest soccer players of all time. In contrast, when the founder of Netflix went to Blockbuster, Blockbuster didn't buy the story. We all know how that turned out. The Blockbuster Video store in our suburb became a relic but I flick on Netflix all the time.

That's not to say that business isn't based on intelligence. Money is one of the greatest motivators of human activity. To this end, I was constantly surprised at how comprehensive business intelligence could be. I have a friend who works for a global advertising company. They can get information on everything from people's communications habits to their locations to the nature of social contacts all through the data sold from their free email accounts. It's all there, easily accessible.

Still, all of that is often not helpful if you can't tell the right story.

For that reason, the business world relies on good communication. If you want to sell a product, you need to hit the target audience. Your communication has to be perfect. It has to speak the right language. The tone needs to be just so. The imagery needs to touch the heart. Otherwise, you've wasted millions of dollars. When we talk about Ferrari, Louis Vuitton, Coca-Cola, McDonald's or Qantas, nothing more needs to be said. We know what each of those brands stand for. That's been achieved through years of effective communication. Remember the Old Spice ads?

Stepping into these worlds taught me some important lessons, because I realised that science could learn a thing or two from business. The scientific world is often terrible at communicating. Most scientists expect the public to celebrate their work because the merit is thought to be inherent. But they don't tell the story – they get into the technical aspects of their work without much thought to the audience. Their presentations are filled with jargon. Media appearances leave people befuddled. Papers are inde-cipherable – even to fellow professionals.

In 2020, I was in a meeting with a bunch of academics. They worked in the same research group, carrying out projects in the same discipline. They were asked to give the government a presentation about their work with the goal of getting some funding. However, some academics from this group were going to be absent when the presentation was scheduled. They were debating how to manage the situation. They were worried about how to describe all the projects.

'Can't one of you just explain your absent colleague's work?' I asked.

'We can't explain the work the other person is doing,' one said.

'Why not?'

'It's too complicated. We don't really understand each other's work.'

Wait. They don't understand each other's work, but they expect the outside world to understand it? They expect government decision-makers to award funding for work that not even they can understand?

Between 2017 and 2018, a group carried out a study where 20 bogus papers were submitted to peer-reviewed academic journals. The exercise became known as the Grievance Studies Affair. Seven out of the 20 papers were accepted at one point. Four of those were published. They had titles like 'An Ethnography of Breastaurant Masculinity: Themes of Objectification, Sexual Conquest, Male Control, and Masculine Toughness in a Sexually Objectifying Restaurant'. Utter nonsense, on purpose. While not accepted immediately, four papers with titles like 'Stars, Planets, and Gender: A Framework for a Feminist Astronomy' were returned to be revised and resubmitted. Although the papers were solely based on sociology, it still highlights how indecipherably dense communication can be in academia.

There's a fallacy in scientific disciplines in the belief that complexity means sophistication. I know a professor who loved to say that 'if we don't demonstrate how complex our work is, people won't realise how much effort goes into it'. This approach leads to complex language, lengthy presentations and distracting communication that loses an audience. I've been in meetings where million-dollar funding opportunities have been lost through this misguided thinking. I could pinpoint the moment where the audience lost interest and the deal was lost.

The famous investor Peter Lynch says never to invest in an idea that you can't illustrate with a crayon. While the heart of that message is about investing in simple things, it also demonstrates why communicating simply is important. We need to understand each other's ideas, no matter what background we are from. And what's more, simplicity is the ultimate form of sophistication as another great, Leonardo da Vinci, said. That's why the greatest scientists are also brilliant communicators. Albert Einstein. Neil deGrasse Tyson. Bill Nye. Carl Sagan. Stephen Hawking. They all communicated so well with us mere mortals.

The lessons I learned about communicating from working at Triad have been invaluable for my work as a doctor and scientist. These days, I make an effort to explain our scientific ventures in the simplest language – not just to the general public, but to my colleagues. The details can follow depending on the audience and level of interest.

Much of the critical communication I did at Triad was about getting a point across under pressure. It wasn't unusual for me and the team to sit in front of a senior government minister, chief executive officer, or other high-level decision-maker. We had to communicate an idea clearly in a brief period of time, snagging their interest. I was generally in charge of communicating strategy – that is, explaining why an idea will work. This included statistics, both good and bad precedents, market data, and an argument about why our idea is what the public may want. After my little presentation, the creative team took over to explain how a strategic idea would come to life. They described the visuals, colours and narratives. In the advertising world, this is called a pitch.

The pitch was always exciting. After getting a brief from a client to make a pitch, multiple advertising agencies battled for their business. The team built up to it over many weeks, throwing ideas around in a creative hotpot. Ideas could change at the last minute. We took new directions. We stayed up late. Finally, everything was ready. After making the pitch, it felt like a whole heap of steam was blown off. Sometimes, we won the client, but of course, sometimes we lost. It was fun.

I didn't realise it then, but I was starting to come alive again. I was becoming energised. In the fondest way, Sarva sometimes likes to say that he had created a monster. This was the start.

That's how this doctor, lawyer, researcher and disability advocate spent a couple of years in advertising. It still feels surreal that I went from being a critically injured patient in an Australian hospital, to struggling through life in Sri Lanka, to finding a temporary career in the world of business. It goes to show that no matter where you are, there's often an opportunity to learn something valuable and grow from it.

My mindset started to shift around then. The philosopher Seneca said, 'Do not seek to have events happen as you want them to, but instead want them to happen as they do happen, and your life will go well.' Leading on from this line of thought is the stoic principle, *amor fati*. Love what happens to you.

I began to love what happened to me. I understood that it gave me the opportunity to grow in ways that I could have never imagined. I was growing into a better person than I might have been if the accident didn't happen. Life became better.

After getting back on our feet, so to speak, Mum and I moved into a new apartment building. It was a modern open-plan apartment full of light. We had great views of Colombo. Having spent many months of my life holed up in a hospital, I've craved living spaces that are connected to the world. I don't close the blinds. I leave doors and windows open as much as possible. Our apartment in Colombo was wrapped in glass all the way around. It was perfect. Although, one flaw was that the designers evidently hadn't accounted for heat expansion and contraction. When the sun hit the building through the day, the windows occasionally spontaneously exploded. Still, it was a great place to live.

One day, I jumped into the lift with a lanky blond guy. I said hello. He replied in a thick Swedish accent. This was Alex, a Swedish entrepreneur who worked for an investment bank. The bank built classifieds websites in developing nations, and Alex was running the Sri Lankan one. It had quickly become the biggest website in the country. He was also selling formal dresses globally online, which was a promising business.

Alex and I became friends. We often met up at the nearby hotel, where we ate together and shared stories about Sweden and Australia. We had great conversations about business. His entrepreneurial spirit was strong.

We spoke about the boom of mobile devices in Sri Lanka. A lot of Sri Lankans were coming online and were hungry for content. However, there was very little Sri Lankan language content for them to consume in those days. Over a beer, we hatched an idea. We were inspired by the website BuzzFeed, which provides random interesting content for people. It was big. We decided to replicate that exact concept in the local language. 'Make it super simple, not complicated,' Alex always said. His approach was quintessentially Scandinavian. Clean. Minimalistic.

I built the website myself. We called it Yako. 'Yako' means devil, but the word is used to indicate surprise as well. As soon as we launched the site, it took off. We kept releasing interesting articles on various topics. They were simple things like, 'The ten most expensive desserts you can buy'. The feedback was great and the traffic grew quickly.

Good business ideas come out of one thing – addressing a need. It's that simple. Sri Lankans just wanted content in the local language.

Sri Lanka and its growing economy had many needs and a huge appetite for new things. For that reason, entrepreneurship was booming. Those days, most of the time, you could just replicate a good idea from a developed country and it took off.

I met some other fascinating entrepreneurs too. One of the most interesting was Merrill J Fernando. Merrill was the founder of the tea company, Dilmah. We met and chatted over a cup of tea, unsurprisingly. He started the company at age 58. 58! He's someone who teaches us that it is never too late to chase a dream. Dilmah is now a world-renowned company. The product is available in over 100 countries as of 2022. Apart from the runaway success that he created, what I found most striking about Merrill was that he was a quiet giver. Ten per cent of pre-tax profits from his companies go to a charitable foundation that aims to help people across the country. Unlike the woman who thought that people living in poverty are sinners, apparently a view shared by some of Merrill's wealthy business colleagues, Merrill specifically said in an interview that he disagrees with this assumption. Merrill has done an impressive amount of socially responsible work without making too much fuss about it. He hasn't got away quietly though, being awarded the Oslo Business for Peace Award for his efforts in 2015.

Even though I was getting back into a working life, the spinal cord injury still caused some medical issues. I was still in the early stages after the injury, which put me at risk for some complications.

One night, I woke up feeling like my heart was racing. I felt my pulse. It was quick. I was short of breath. Every time I tried to take a deep breath, my left shoulder tip hurt. I felt ill. We phoned a house-call doctor who came and examined me. 'You're anxious,' they said. 'You're probably just depressed from the accident.' They left. I tried not to be my own doctor. After all, I'd only just made it to the third year of medical school at that point. *Fine*, I thought. *Maybe it's just anxiety*. Though uncomfortable, I went back to sleep.

The next day, I felt faint after getting up, and then I passed out. Mum and my then assistant laid me flat. I regained consciousness shortly afterwards. I thought that this was just physical deconditioning. I used to pass out a lot back in the spinal unit. So, I ignored it and kept going about my business. From then on, however, I kept getting shortness of breath, shoulder tip pain and a racing heart. Over the days that followed, it became more and more frequent. I consulted a couple of other doctors, but they all said the same thing: 'It's anxiety.'

One night, the symptoms became so bad that I closely listened to my chest with my stethoscope. On the left side, I could hear what's called a pleural rub. It was loud. A pleural rub is a coarse sound like sandpaper rubbing together. It can be a sign of some pretty bad things in my context, so again I consulted a doctor.

'I listened to my chest here and I can hear a pleural rub,' I told them.

'I can't hear anything. I think you're just anxious,' was the doctor's curt response. Surprise.

As more days went by, the symptoms worsened. I started to faint all the time. I couldn't ignore it now; I was really concerned. In particular, I was worried that I had a pulmonary embolism. This is a blood clot that travels to the lung from the leg. People with spinal cord injuries can be at risk of them, particularly in the early stages of an injury. I knew there was a blood test that could rule it out called a D-dimer. I finally managed to talk to someone who requested the test – and it was positive. This doctor immediately requested a CT scan to look for a blood clot, and while none was found, the test did show up a large amount of fluid around my left lung. The fluid was taking up more than half the chest cavity.

I was admitted to the hospital straight away. I was relieved that we found an answer. I was relieved that it was being taken seriously. The doctors inserted a drain, and the fluid that drained away was suggestive of something sinister in the lung cavity – maybe even a cancer, I was told. I thought, *Really? After all this, there's now something nasty in my chest?*

The plan was to do a thoracoscopy next. This allows doctors to look inside the chest cavity to see what's there. A doctor performed the procedure and found something unusual in the lining of my lung. They were even more worried about something malignant, so a sample was taken and sent to India for analysis. Some of the more sophisticated tests were not available in Sri Lanka. It was going to take a few days for the result to come back.

In the intervening time, I developed a tension pneumothorax. This is when air becomes trapped outside the lung through a one-way valve in the chest wall. The procedures that were performed on me had probably left such a one-way valve. The problem with a tension pneumothorax is that air gets sucked into the chest cavity, but it can't escape. As air fills up the chest cavity, it compresses the structures within, including the heart. A tension pneumothorax, when not managed, can be fatal. Once this was discovered, I ended up with another tube in my chest, this one to drain the air.

Unfortunately, the tube caused an infection. I got sepsis – an overwhelming infection that affects the whole body. I was so sick that the doctor talked to me about going on a ventilator. The situation was dire; I was to go back to the intensive care unit, asleep on a ventilator, until I recovered. I couldn't bear the thought.

I begged the doctor to give me time. If I deteriorated more, then I'd go on a ventilator. In retrospect, my choice was an irresponsible one fraught with risk. But, I was just so traumatised by the previous ICU admissions. Luckily, I recovered. I spent several weeks in a Sri Lankan hospital recovering in a normal ward. The results from the lung sample came back in that time. I didn't have cancer.

In the next year or two, I spent a cumulative three or four months in hospital over a number of stays with different complications. The hospital staff got to know me well.

I was on the verge of death more than once. One day, I again developed autonomic dysreflexia. It was because of urinary retention. We knew exactly what needed to be done but needed a hospital urgently. Mum called an ambulance, but while we waited for it, my blood pressure crept up. It started to reach levels that were concerning for causing a stroke or something severe. My heart rate started to drop.

When I got to the hospital, I was met by a young doctor. He didn't know what autonomic dysreflexia was. For situations like this, my mum had a card displaying a printed explanation. These cards are easily accessible on the internet for patients to carry around, because autonomic dysreflexia is not widely known. The cards explain how to diagnose and treat it, and they also highlight the urgency of the condition. She handed the card over to the doctor. He dismissed it. I told him that I was a medical student. I again described what autonomic dysreflexia was.

I explained to him that we needed to drain my bladder urgently to relieve the issue.

'You're just anxious,' he said.

I wasn't just frustrated with his response, I was infuriated.

I was watching the monitor next to my bed. My heart rate was now about 28 beats per minute. The blood pressure was approaching levels that I've never seen in practice – even today. I felt like death. If something wasn't done quickly, I knew that something bad would happen – and probably imminently. Mum got into an argument with the doctor. He was adamant that nothing needed to be done urgently, but that I just needed to calm down. Funny. I've never met an anxious person with a heart rate of 28 beats per minute.

Eventually Mum called Sarva. He arranged for a senior surgeon to rush from another hospital. The surgeon quickly took me to the operating theatre and performed a procedure to address the bladder problem which promptly fixed the autonomic dysreflexia. Blood drained from my bladder for days. The doctor got a proper talking to.

I still try not to be my own doctor. However, these experiences didn't lay a great foundation for that approach. I'm lucky to have the health literacy to be able to navigate these problems. Not everyone has that. Medical training is complex. There is a lot to learn. Always.

Every day, I'm reminded of the Dunning–Kruger effect. This is the tendency to be overconfident about our abilities when we start to learn something new. As we learn more over time, we realise that we actually didn't know much at all. Our confidence takes a hit. Then, as even more time goes by, a much better balance is found between confidence and our level of knowledge. I'm constantly learning how much more there is to know. I'm sure there's an eloquent quote to back me up, but I believe that the cornerstone of wisdom is knowing that we don't know everything.

So, how do we walk this line between being a medical expert and empowering the patient? In my view, a lot of it simply lies in listening to the patient. We need to understand their concerns. We need to work collaboratively. Paternalism isn't the way.

Imagine if the doctor had listened to me. Imagine if he had taken the card and given it some thought. Imagine if the other doctors hadn't immediately thought that I was just anxious. Maybe the pleural effusion would've been diagnosed sooner to prevent the subsequent train wreck of further complications.

Again, they say to 'listen to the customer' in the business world. Mahatma Gandhi is sometimes credited with saying, 'A customer is the most important visitor on our premises, he is not dependent on us. We are dependent on him. He is not an interruption in our work. He is the purpose of it. He is not an outsider in our business. He is part of it. We are not doing him a favor by serving him. He is doing us a favor by giving us an opportunity to do so.' Although this philosophy is used widely in teaching customer service, there are clear parallels to medicine as well. Our patients are the purpose of our work.

Back to the train wreck. Ego also probably played some part in all this. Many doctors have big egos. I must say, disability plays some part in it too. People with disabilities generally have a different healthcare experience from their counterparts without disability. There's a health gap between people with disabilities and those without. There's a difference in life expectancy. There are differences again between developed and developing nations.

The situation for many people with spinal cord injuries in Sri Lanka is grim. There's a spinal injuries unit in Colombo. When I visited to see how I could help out, I found an area about 20 metres by 5 metres. There were basic flat hospital beds lined up on either side of the room. There was one bathroom. There was no climate control, which would've made things difficult for the patients, many of whom couldn't control their body temperature. There was little equipment and minimal resources. The occasional stray cat roamed around the unit.

I'm not trying to disparage the place. The country had precious few resources, and allocating them was tough. These are just the circumstances that people lived with, and the staff did the best they could.

One of the patients had been in the unit for months. He had developed a pressure ulcer. These can be common in people with spinal cord injuries. With paralysis, there is no sensation to the areas that are under pressure from the body's weight. If those areas remain under pressure even for a couple of hours, the skin starts to break down. The person doesn't feel pain, so they don't move around to relieve the pressure. The pressure continues to damage the skin. Eventually, an ulcer forms. This particular patient's pressure ulcer was so bad that it had eaten through to one of the large bones in the leg, causing infection. The bone had to be replaced with a prosthetic.

Too many of the patients from that unit went home, never to be heard of again. 'They sadly perish,' a doctor said. These were rural folk. There was no comprehensive medical care where they lived. Social support was scarce. These injuries were sometimes taboo. Life was often short.

After seeing all this, I counted my blessings every day. My life was a stark contrast to some of the people I saw. When I was well and out of hospital, I was rolling around Colombo eating at the best restaurants and hanging out at the nicest locations. Sarva introduced me to people and I made friends. Many of them were impressive. Some were captains of industry, others were politicians or prominent artists.

One day I went to a party at someone's house. There, I met a beautiful woman. We'll call her Coco. She had flawless skin, beautiful eyes and a girlish demeanour. She was fun. Coco was a well-known artist. After we met briefly that night, we went our separate ways.

A few weeks later, I turned up at a restaurant after work to grab some dinner. The restaurant was inside an old colonial building turned hotel in the middle of Colombo. There was no one in the restaurant except Coco. Again, we said hello, ate a meal separately, then took off.

A few weeks after that, I was sitting at my favourite café in Colombo having breakfast. I was at my preferred table closest to the main road, reading a newspaper. The sun was shining. I was loving life. Then, a passing car pulled over and a woman jumped out and walked up to the café. She approached me and said, 'Hi, do you remember me? It's Coco.'

'Yes! I remember. How are you?' I replied.

'I'm really good. I have to run back to the car, but let's catch up sometime?' She gave me her number then took off.

We started talking on the phone. We texted each other all the time. We hung out every now and again. I liked her.

Coco loved Marilyn Monroe. She also loved white chocolate KitKats. If I ever saw them, I got her some. She loved the Of Monsters and Men song, 'Little Talks'. Every time I hear it now, I'm reminded of Coco.

One day, we were texting each other when she typed, *I'm hooked.*

What do you mean? I said.

I'm hooked on you.

After that, we were briefly close. She used to do shout-outs to me on TV, where she had her own show. We had the occasional little fight. I remember one of them clearly for what we said, but not what it was about.

'You're such an ass,' she said.

'Yeah, but I'm a cute ass,' I replied.

'You're so annoying. But, yes.'

Knowing my love of cars, Coco organised for me to go for a spin in a Lamborghini for my 29th birthday. The car was driven by a skilled race driver who had won several cups. His white Lamborghini was an amazing car. It had some customisations that were unique; Lamborghini had made this car specially for him. It wasn't easy to get into, but with some help I managed to stuff myself into it. The interior was relatively bare – some luxuries had been removed to save weight. This machine was made for speed.

The driver turned on the engine. As the engine was in the rear, its sound boomed behind my head. He drove expertly out of the building into the main streets of Colombo, and from there he started to pump it. The engine noise was explosive. The car handled like it was on rails. My body took all the forces as a result. I held on. When he hit the brakes, the seatbelts engaged to stop my body flying forward. As we sped through the narrow streets of the small city, the policemen waved. They were too scared to stop anyone that wealthy. It was easily the most raw, brutal, exhilarating driving experience I have ever had.

I'm not sure what happened, but after a little while Coco and I suddenly stopped talking. That was it. I stopped hearing from her. Nonetheless, it was my first experience of being emotionally close to anyone, years after Yaris.

Sometimes, people fleetingly cross each other's paths. It can be brief and bright, like two shooting stars colliding, but just as quickly, the fire sometimes burns out. And that's okay. The memory of that explosion can last a lifetime. As they say, it's not about the number of breaths you take. It's about the number of moments that take your breath away. I've been lucky enough to have a life filled with moments that took my breath away.

As I ventured out into the world more, my sense of self began to come back. I started looking in the mirror again – maybe even a little too much. I started dressing better. I got my hair cut properly. For the longest time, I had worn fur-lined foot covers that the spinal injuries unit made for their patients. I started wearing proper shoes instead. I actually have a thing for shoes. I have a thing for watches too. I treated myself to a decent watch.

This time, my sense of self was a bit different. I didn't really care what the outside world thought. I was comfortable within myself. What I did for myself was just to make me happy.

There is an epidemic of low self-esteem in the world. I think it's partly because people seek validation from outside to inform their self-worth. Traditional and social media portray idealised lifestyles and body images that are neither real nor truly the definition of happiness. What we see is just a snapshot of a person's life. That snapshot only shows us the outside of that person, too. These images lead us to believe that our lives are less than ideal. They beckon us to believe that we are less, because our lives don't match the highlight reels that others portray on screens. This causes high levels of loneliness, envy, anxiety, depression and narcissism, resulting in a world where suicide is the leading cause of death globally for 15–29-year-olds in 2021. People are getting hurt.

I dated a woman on and off for a couple of years in my early 20s. She was beautiful. She'd been through many challenges as a kid. She occasionally struggled with depression. In her early 20s, she was really into pop culture. She loved Paris Hilton, and bought a dog just like Paris's dog. She bought handbags and phones that celebrities had. Her career plans aligned with whatever movie she was watching that week. In *How to Lose a Guy in Ten Days*, Kate Hudson played a journalist. So she wanted to be a journalist. In *Nip/Tuck*, the main characters were plastic surgeons. So she wanted to be a plastic surgeon. At one point, her sole goal was just to be a wealthy socialite. She was never happy.

She's a lovely person, and she's doing well now. But over a decade later, she told me, 'If only I'd known then what I know now.' Sometimes, the wrong influence can eat up a critical part of a person's life. But it's not just the media consumer who's at risk. Creators can be too.

Over time, I've met people who are media personalities. I've noticed that for some, their sense of self-worth is drawn from the outside world. Validation comes from fans celebrating them. The irony. Fans look at their icon's lives thinking that it's idyllic. It's a damaging cycle where no one realises the truth.

One of my senior colleagues used to talk about 'inward-looking broken people'. According to my colleague, these are people who always need to fill their cup without much thought about anyone else. They focus on their needs alone. They only think about their problems. They fail to look outside themselves.

After 37 short years on this planet, the most important thing I've learned is that looking inwards is like looking into a bottomless pit. A black hole. It's a never-ending vacuum that requires constant attention. It's the reason why we want more likes on social media. It's the reason why we seek outside validation. It's the reason that we distract ourselves with possessions, social status and titles. But here's the secret. True happiness comes from looking outwards. Happiness is about compassion. Empathy. Giving. By giving ourselves to the outside world, we paradoxically feel complete. That's why the happiest people on earth are givers, not takers.

Deep.

After a while, I started to feel complete again. I was living a pretty good life in Sri Lanka. I was comfortable.

Mum was doing well. We had a solid support network. We felt at home.

After a great deal of effort, Sarva convinced me to go to the cinema for the first time since the accident. It had been a couple of years since I sat in front of the big screen. We watched *The Avengers*. On occasion, he took me to parties. To have a group of overconfident drunk people carry a wheelchair up three flights of stairs wrapping around the outside of a building with no handrails to get to a rooftop party was certainly a thrill. Let me tell you, Colombo can really party.

I had some other unique experiences too. One time, I was doing a talk at a prominent health event in Sri Lanka. In the audience was a policymaker. After the talk, he came over to me.

'I would love to chat to you about some things. Would you like to come to my office?' he said.

Relishing the opportunity to talk about Sri Lankan health policy, I went to his office. It was tucked away on the ground floor of a government building. He asked everyone else to leave the room. Mum must have got bored waiting outside, because when I looked out the window I saw her driving off. Presumably, she thought that I would catch up later. I was alone in the room with the bureaucrat. The doors were shut. There was an odd silence.

'Let me move closer to you,' the bureaucrat said in a somewhat sensual tone.

He moved very close so that we were nearly touching.

'You know, I'm married for appearances. But, I also have an alternative lifestyle. I keep a separate apartment for rendezvous. Shall we go there right now?' he continued.

He started to move even closer.

'Uhhh . . . guys, let's go!' I yelled out.

My assistant ran in. I made a rapid exit.

There's a bit to unpack from that experience, but that brazen attempt to take advantage of me made me wonder how many people that bureaucrat had done this to. It's another reminder that people with disabilities disproportionally experience all kinds of violence, including sexual harassment. It only takes a quick internet search to find some harrowing stories.

Even though I was enjoying life again in Colombo, I was thinking about medical school every day. It was still my dream to be a doctor. It was a dream that beckoned again and again. My brief career in advertising had been fun and rewarding, but my heart looked to medicine. I just knew it was where I belonged.

Have you ever read *The Alchemist* by Paulo Coelho? The book has sold over 65 million copies as I write this. It spent over 300 weeks on the *New York Times* bestseller list. Its success is one thing, but what is great about the book are the lessons within.

In a nutshell, the story is about a young lad who dreams of finding treasure. He embarks upon a journey, experiencing many things along the way, like hardship. In the end, it turns out that the treasure was back home where he started the whole time.

To me, the story tells us that the journey is what's most important – not the destination. The journey is where we learn and grow. And sometimes, the treasure ends up being back where we started. We had it all along. But, if it weren't for the journey, we wouldn't know that the treasure was there. Medicine was like that for me.

As I pondered all this, time moved on. It was 2014. I had the accident in 2010. In mid-2014, academics from the medical school were having regular remote meetings with me. 'If you want to come back, now is the time,' they said. Soon, it'll be too late, and my chance would be gone.

Around that time, I also explored what medical schools were like for people with disabilities in Sri Lanka. Only one medical school was open to the conversation. All the other schools thought that it was a ridiculous idea. How could a doctor with quadriplegia work?

I had conversations with friends about what to do next. Some suggested that I keep doing the work I was doing. Some suggested that I work as a lawyer. I had some tempting offers to build a career in Sri Lanka in business or law.

Here's the thing. In life, many people will have an opinion about what you should and shouldn't do. Always.

Many years from now, though, you'll be at the end of the road looking back. You'll take stock of the journey. At that point, there'll only be one person you can hold responsible for the choices you made – and that's you. It's not your teacher or your boss. It's not society. It's not a movie, or a celebrity. It's not the school bully. It's not your controlling partner. None of those other people will be there. If you're going to listen to others, you'd better know for sure that it's the right choice for you.

One day, you'll be the only person left who you can hold accountable for your life.

I knew that if I didn't come back to Australia to take my place in medical school, I'd regret it forever. Marcus Aurelius said, 'Remember how long you've been putting this off, how many extensions the gods gave you, and you didn't use them. At some point you have to recognise what the world it is that you belong to; what power rules it and from what source you spring; that there is a limit to the time assigned to you, and if you don't use it to free yourself it will be gone and will never return.'

I couldn't bear the idea of my chance never returning. Even though the overwhelming majority of people told me that I shouldn't, I wanted to try.

I spoke to Mum. We knew that it would be hard, but 'Let's do it,' she said. She didn't even think twice. She was ready to give up our comforts to help me pursue the dream.

I also spoke to Sarva.

'I'm going to go and try,' I said.

'You're not going to try. If you're going to go, go and kick ass. There is no try,' he said.

Sri Lanka healed my soul. It gave me back my sense of self. I was strong again.

It was time to circle back, to pick up the treasure where I left it.

6

THE PATIENT MEDICAL STUDENT

Every difficulty in life presents us with an opportunity to turn inward and to invoke our own inner resources. The trials we endure can and should introduce us to our strengths . . . Dig deeply. You possess strengths you might not realise you have.

Epictetus

MUM AND I came back to Brisbane in November 2014. We started life again with next to nothing. Although we accumulated some comforts in Sri Lanka, there was still little of significance to bring back with us. We only had some bags and a wheelchair. And well, the airline broke the wheelchair.

Settling in was a bit easier than it might have been thanks to some help. This is where my supervisor from the very first rotation in medical school, psychiatry, came back into my life.

Harry McConnell went to a great deal of trouble to help me navigate my return to medical school. While many were supportive, Harry told me he had backroom conversations with some who were sceptical. He apparently had to convince them that it would be a worthwhile exercise to take me back. On top of that, Harry worked on setting up some social support, engaging a social organisation to secure a small apartment containing the bare essentials for Mum and me. We also organised some support staff to help me.

After landing in Australia, Mum and I jumped straight into the business of setting up life. This included the basics, like buying a toaster and having the internet connected. The journey back to medical school was going to happen quickly – we landed in late November, and I was to start in January.

I was to be a student at the Gold Coast University Hospital. At one point in the 2010s, this was one of the most expensive hospitals ever built in human history. It was an impressive building. The hospital often gives me pause to think about life in an economically prosperous country. This hospital, with its state-of-the-art architecture, equipment and medical care, offers the public free healthcare. Free! There are billions of people on this planet who don't have anywhere near such a luxury.

The first step was meeting with the dean of the medical school, Professor Simon Broadley. He was a neurologist with expertise in multiple sclerosis who had trained in England. He was well spoken and the sort of person I always imagined the quintessential English gentleman to be. Although he jokingly told me never to tell anyone, the medical students of old called him 'The Broadsword' in reference to his name and leadership status.

'Of course, there's no question that we'll have you back,' he said. However, Professor Broadley asked me whether I was sure that this was what I wanted. He asked whether I understood that this journey would be difficult. My answer was clear: yes, I understood that it was going to be challenging. Still, I wanted to come back.

The next step was to meet the doctors who were to supervise me over the next two years. I was at the point where there was little classroom activity, but lots of learning within the hospital.

I met a spectrum of personalities, many of them welcoming. The surgeon was an Austrian who was fond of Arnold Schwarzenegger. He was friendly, but truly surgical in our discussion – to the point. The obstetrician and gynaecologist was warm. She was of South African origin. The psychiatrist was quirky with an enormous intellect and a lush head of brush-like hair, and the nephrologist extremely clever and stoic.

Someone from another specialty, however, was less optimistic. I later heard that they'd said things like, 'I don't know if patients will take him seriously'. They never said anything untoward to my face, but persisted in making comments behind the scenes.

Then, I met the emergency physician, Dr Lauren Stephenson. We met in the hospital lobby. Lauren was caring, warm. She said hello to my mum. She bought us coffee. We sat down at a table outside and Lauren asked me questions about my life. She had a great deal of empathy for what had happened to me. 'We'll make it work,' she said finally. As soon as she said that, I knew that we really would.

Doctors like Lauren work in dynamic environments. Things change rapidly and chaos regularly ensues. They face different scenarios all the time. It could be anything from a trauma to a heart attack, a drug overdose or a drowning. They are often interrupted. There are in fact studies observing one interruption about every six minutes for a doctor working in an emergency department. This seems realistic, because one of my colleagues once counted 129 interruptions during a 10.5-hour shift.

With this going on in the background, these doctors manage teams in the most difficult circumstances. Therefore, they need to have a collected leadership style in the thick of a storm. Shaped by all that, the ones I met up till that point had a calm, relaxed confidence about them, just like Lauren. Maybe that's why I trusted what she said.

After I got the go-ahead from all of my supervisors, I set about the task of learning how to do things again. The medical school secured some resources to obtain a teacher and an actor to play the patient. This way, I had the opportunity to problem-solve ways of doing things on a one-on-one basis. We had many sessions together over a number of weeks. In those sessions, I learned how to hold a stethoscope. I learned how to examine a patient. All of it was exciting, but sometimes painstaking.

I also learned how to do procedures with the help of an intensive care nurse called Jenny. One day, we sat down with a cannula. This is a metallic needle surrounded by a rubber-like flexible translucent tube. The cannula is inserted into a vein through the skin. The rubber-like tube is left in while the needle is pulled out. That tube can be used to deliver fluids or medications into the patient's vein. After the accident, I never thought that I would be able to insert a cannula, but after Jenny and I messed around with a cannula for hours one day, I eventually succeeded in putting one into a model vein. While this is a simple procedure that doctors, nurses, paramedics, and the guys in that dark dodgy park down the street do every single day, it was a giant step for me.

Attitudes alone are the biggest barriers to achieving things: not only the attitudes of other people, but attitudes within ourselves. I thought that I'd never be able to perform simple procedures. Yet, here I was putting in a cannula. I was more able than I imagined. I just had to try. As I achieved these small successes, other people around me started to change their attitude too. Pessimism was giving way to optimism, albeit slowly.

I was put in touch with my predecessor, Dr Harry Eeman, who went through medical school using a wheelchair due to Guillain-Barré syndrome. Harry and I often spent time talking about how to do medical school from the wheelchair while managing a complex life. It was good to have someone who had trod this path before. Harry gave me plenty of tips. We became good friends.

The days plodded along. Christmas came. Mum and I were alone, but happy.

This is probably a good spot to note that people often ask me why I don't talk about my half-sister and father. The truth is, I haven't seen or heard from them for many years. The trauma that my family went through pulled us apart. They'll have their own versions of why they didn't remain a part of this journey.

What I can say is that difficult times test the strength of the bonds in families. Sometimes, they break. And that's okay. Sometimes, they become stronger than ever to shine brighter than ever. Stars are fuelled this way too, you know. A huge amount of force can push two atoms together to release an incredible amount of energy. It's how our sun exists.

I focus on the stars that were formed, for these are the ones that light up my life every day. The others have faded into the night. Just like the unseen stars, they have no impact on my life. But the brightest star is my mum.

Anyway, we had a simple Christmas that year. No celebration, no other family, and not much else. On New Year's Eve,

Mum and I were still alone in the apartment. At about 9 pm that night, Mum was cleaning up some old paperwork and came across a police report from my accident. The report had a mobile number for the person who pulled over, held my bleeding head, and waited for emergency services – Chris Bailey. I took a chance. I sent a text message to the mobile number.

Hi, I wonder if you remember pulling over for a guy in a car accident in January 2010? my message said.

Not long afterwards, I got a reply. *Can I call you?*

Chris called me. He was at a New Year's Eve party. The whole party stopped – everyone was listening to our conversation. They were enthralled by the story.

It turns out that Chris had desperately tried to look for me after that night. Because of privacy reasons, no one had told him what happened to me. He even placed an advertisement in the newspaper but never found out what happened. To get a text message from me was a huge surprise.

We shared our memories of what had happened that night. I told him about my journey from that point, and Chris told me about his life. We were like long-lost family reconnecting. A bond like the one we made in those fateful minutes lasts forever. We talked for more than an hour and promised to stay connected.

In January 2015, I was ready to come back to medical school. The official start date was in the middle of January. The day quickly approached, but I was nervous.

Two days before I was due to start, I began feeling a little bit off. I went to the GP, who did a urine test. The next day, she called me. She was concerned that I had a urinary tract infection, and she wanted me to go to the emergency department. I asked if there was anything else that we could do, but no. I must go to the emergency department for antibiotics through a drip, she said.

Reluctantly, I arrived at the same hospital where I was only days away from starting as a medical student. I was put into an emergency bed. The team got a cannula into me and delivered antibiotics through it. Fortunately, I didn't have to stay longer than a few hours.

Finally, the kick-off day arrived. After five years away, I sat in an auditorium for the orientation covering the clinical students starting that year. The faces were all unfamiliar. They looked young. When I initially started medical school, the average starting age for students was something like 24. In the five years I'd been away, this age had dropped dramatically due to changes in the entry pathway. I felt like an outsider. Not only was I coming into the company of complete strangers, but I was in a different physical state to them – in a wheelchair. I sat in the front of the auditorium in the space made for a wheelchair user, feeling even more awkward.

Professor Broadley welcomed the class into their clinical years. He made a brief diversion to introduce me, and asked everyone to make me feel welcome. During a break later that day, a student came up to me. Her name was

Christina, and she told me that she was an intensive care nurse before getting into medical school. Seeing me there was quite something for her, because apparently she looked after me in the intensive care unit after the accident. I didn't remember her but was blown away by the coincidence.

My first rotation was psychiatry, which made me feel like I was picking up where I left off. In reality, the specialty was chosen for me because of the pace. There's no need to run around. There's less chaos – at least most of the time. Nonetheless, psychiatry is fascinating. It's one of the frontiers of medicine. There are many undiscovered things about how the mind works. More and more, we are unravelling the interactions between our biological and psychological self.

For example, it's hypothesised that hormonal changes following stress causes Takotsubo cardiomyopathy or 'broken-heart syndrome'. In this condition, the heart is physically affected as a result of a stressful event. It's a real thing that we see in the hospital. Similarly, some researchers write that happiness is associated with a longer life and better health. There are also links between exercise, diet and mental health. While the biological interactions behind all this are complex, I know that happiness is a big part of why I feel physically well.

The comparatively slower pace of psychiatry was an opportunity to troubleshoot things like what to wear. With a spinal cord injury, the lower limbs can swell quickly. If my shoes are too tight, the swelling can cause wounds at pressure points. Autonomic dysreflexia can occur because of pain in the feet. I tried a bunch of different professional shoes until we found something that worked. It was the same case with clothes. Tight pants can quickly cause problems. Finding something suitable took a bit of trial and error.

Before I came back to medical school, I often talked to my schoolfriend Dean about it. He had a great deal of advice that I always valued, but one of the things that resonated with me was when he suggested that I think about this situation as though I were an athlete, because I was breaking new ground. 'If you want to perform well, you're going to need to be disciplined like an Olympian,' said Dean. I took his advice to heart. Dean was right. If I was to make it work, I needed to treat life with an athlete's attitude. In addition to his sage advice, Dean gave me a chunk of money to get started again. He's always been like that. Dean looks after everyone around him.

Dean wasn't the only one who made me think about performance. The philosopher Epictetus once said, 'The true man is revealed in difficult times. So when trouble comes, think of yourself as a wrestler whom God, like a trainer, has paired with a tough young buck. For what purpose? To turn you into Olympic-class material.' After I spoke at a conference one day, an orthopaedic surgeon pulled me aside for a chat. She told me about the gender barriers that she had to fight to get where she was. Disability is like that too, she said. 'Your life is one where you need to think about high performance. Your dreams, your work, they all rely on high performance. Make sure you structure your life to get every inch of performance that you can to prove yourself,' she concluded.

It's true, isn't it? High performance is about eking out every inch. On 31 May 2008, Usain Bolt broke the world record for the hundred-metre sprint. His speed was 9.72 seconds. His predecessor, Asafa Powell, held the previous record at 9.74 seconds. Two-hundredths of a second. That's all it was. As soon as Usain Bolt shaved off that extra 0.02 seconds, his name went down in the history books.

I learned that the pursuit of excellence is also founded in humility. That's because we need humility to be acquainted with our weaknesses. I noticed that people who excel at things are often more interested in what their weaknesses are than their strengths. This is not in a self-denigrating way, but as part of a never-ending quest to become better. Dean once told me, 'I love it when people tell me when I can improve.' It's probably why he's one of the best doctors that I know. Weaknesses are a challenge, and challenges are good. Otherwise, there is no growth. I, too, started focusing on my weaknesses. I wanted to challenge myself.

For example, I hated ECGs or electrocardiograms when I was in medical school before the accident. An ECG is the tracing of the electrical activity in the heart. You can use them to diagnose important things like a heart attack or an abnormal rhythm. I hated them. Wanting to challenge myself, I decided to throw as many ECGs as I could at me. Eventually, I became more comfortable with them.

In our efforts to become better, Mum and I worked on making a streamlined process for me to get ready in the morning. Even with this process, I got up 3.5 hours before I was due somewhere. My friend Jesse introduced me to the concept of a positive morning routine. 'It's important to start your day with positive thoughts,' he told me. Jesse sent me a bunch of motivational soundtracks to have playing in the background when I woke up. These were full of messages that kept me fired up. 'Stay hungry,' the motivational speaker Les Brown screamed. 'If you want it, work,' an unknown speaker yelled. This was the soundtrack for the first hour.

In that first hour, Mum helped me with breakfast, brushing my teeth and those little things. After that, she got herself ready while I did administrative bits like email, bills and things of that nature on my laptop. At that point, a support person came to the house to help. We went to the shower, jumped back in the bed, got dressed, popped back to the wheelchair, then Mum and I ran to the tram. In the tram, we kept warm with a coffee on the way to the hospital. While this routine sounds simple, the logistics required teamwork. I couldn't just get up and walk into the shower. Showering required help. Dressing required help. We timed everything to the minute. We refined parts of the process, such as putting on socks a certain way to make it quicker. We turned into a finely tuned machine.

At the start of being back at medical school, Mum and I didn't have much support. Mum hopped between home and the hospital on the tram to help me through the day. She came to the hospital to help me eat or do other simple personal things, then went back home to go about her business. She was stretched.

Those days, support organisations received state funding to provide services to a person with a disability. But some organisations were predatory. The one I engaged initially gave me no choice about the way support was structured. To maximise profits, they sent staff for most of the day on weekends at high rates – when I needed them the least. Later, we found out they overbilled many people. This particular organisation fell apart, embroiled in controversy, allegations of bad management, and even allegations of mismanagement of sexual abuse incidents involving their clients that were aired in the Royal Commission into Institutional Responses to Child Sexual Abuse (a claim denied by the organisation). When it collapsed, the newspapers had headlines like 'Allegations of bullying, financial malpractice', 'Boss of charity that made a $5.2 million loss is criticised for taking three staff on a 12,000 km trip to Africa to lecture women about business – complete with a champagne dinner to kick off' and 'Queensland boss attacks "slovenly" and "toxic" employees in LinkedIn post'.

Mum eventually learned to navigate the systems. She advocated to have support structured the way we needed it.

To ensure that an unknown organisation could not take control of my life, she managed everything. We learned to hire our own staff, people who we bonded with. We worked out how to access equipment like wheelchairs. After learning to help me, Mum's skillset benefited many other people with disabilities, too.

Over time, we built a personal support team that became family. They became affectionately known as 'the boys'. We all shared a single goal – to get me through medical school. We all went for it. We had fun while doing it. We laughed. We joked. This made life as a medical student much easier.

One night, for example, I was at a Brisbane hospital when Dean invited me to spend some time with him. He was the doctor on a night shift. I was the student. I arrived at the car park with one of the boys, Sam. He had a little old red Toyota Corolla. When I slid out from the passenger seat into the wheelchair, my pants came off. It was just Sam and me. There was no one else to help. We tried to figure out the best way to get my pants back on. Eventually, we thought that one way was to open the passenger-side window, throw my torso inside, then have Sam pull up my pants while the legs were hanging out. So, picture this. There was a guy without pants bent over the passenger door of a car, torso inside. There was another guy behind him, standing over him, struggling feverishly to do something. This is what some bystanders ended up seeing that night in the car park of a major hospital. Those were the adventures we had.

The boys helped me with everything from getting around to having a shower. The shower was an oddly productive time. It's where a lot of my inspiration came. I learned a bit of medicine there, too, via medical podcasts that I played while showering. About six years later, I ended up being featured in one of my favourite podcasts, called *Surgery 101*, based in Canada. Knowledge saturation is a great thing. I may not have picked up everything in a podcast, but I often learned one or two pearls. And that was enough. Two pearls a day, six days a week, can add up to over 600 pearls a year. Those pearls regularly came in handy in exams or, more importantly, for patient care.

Speaking of showers, I became acquainted with a very different type of shower too. Spit showers. Evidently, my face is now at the perfect height for people's spit to land on if they are talking passionately. I've noticed that these passions are particularly heightened at events like parties, lubricated by alcohol. I've thought about getting a portable screen that I could hold in front of my face.

Imagine that. 'Excuse me one moment. I want to hear everything you are saying right after I grab this.'

Between coming out of the real shower and hopping into the tram, Mum, my assistant and I switched up the soundtrack. Instead of motivational speakers and medical podcasts, it was upbeat music. The staple was 'Juicy' by The Notorious BIG. So many things about that song resonate with me to this day. Whether you like rap music or not,

'Juicy' is a story about a man who tried to make good from the worst of circumstances. He tried, he succeeded. Everyone around him celebrated. It's a good story. Little did I know just how much of that story would hold true for me in the coming years.

Bouncing off the walls from music and coffee, we arrived in the hospital. I was inevitably rushing as fast as I could to join the ward round. For most specialties, the morning starts with a ward round during which the team reviews all the patients under their care. For each patient, the plan for the next steps is developed.

The ward round is like a line of ducks moving from bed to bed. The hierarchical nature of medicine is reflected in the line of ducks. Even though the order of the line varies, the hierarchy is usually evident from people's behaviour. The seniors are comfortable, relaxed. The juniors are nervous. The layer in between them varies in attitude. The behaviour is a useful measure of a person, because someone once told me that people's attitude while traversing the hierarchy can quickly reveal personality vulnerabilities, especially when they treat others poorly. I agree. For instance, a 2009 paper by Vincent J. Roscigno called 'Supervisory bullying, status inequalities and organizational context' notes that 'bullies may target not only the vulnerable but also those who threaten their sense of superiority or those who make them feel vulnerable'.

On top of the food chain in Australia is the consultant. Everyone defers to them. They're a doctor who has completed all aspects of specialty training. Not only are they a medical expert, but they are responsible for the team and the patients under their care. To become a specialist, it often takes a minimum of six years of further training after medical school for the quickest specialty pathway. Frequently, it will be about 10 years.

Immediately under the consultant is the registrar. There are senior registrars, junior registrars and non-training registrars. They perform a large amount of work, particularly within the public system. They're often decision-makers for things that are not too complex. With the exception of non-training registrars, the other registrars are training to become a specialist. They'll be sitting exams and meeting the various other requirements of whichever training program they are undertaking.

Non-training registrars are ones that are working while trying to get into a specialty. Some specialties are incredibly selective and may only take two or three registrars for the whole country in one year. Non-training registrars may spend years trying to get into these programs. They do courses, buff up their CVs and perform research in their own time. They may also do a tremendous amount of ass-kissing during this time. For entry into many specialties, senior people need to like you.

Below the registrars are residents. Most people spend a couple of years being a resident, then become a registrar of some sort. Residents again can be divided into junior and senior. Residents are doctors with full registration, but they are not specialists. Nor are they on a specialist training program. They may not even have decided what specialty to pursue. Some may have but are waiting to become a registrar.

Then, there's the intern. An intern is just out of medical school. They rotate through a number of core specialties in the space of one year. They are supervised closely and assessed regularly. Interns must pass this year to obtain full registration. For many specialties, interns perform administrative duties. They prepare lists for the ward round, put in requests for various investigations and liaise with other specialties, for example.

Finally, there's the medical student. The bottom of the ladder.

When I came back to medical school, some colleagues from my old class were registrars. Some took the seniority seriously, not wanting to bottom-feed with a lowly student like me.

Remember 'Angus'? He was the guy who I first saw after waking up from the accident. We used to be close. I even once hosted a birthday party for him in my apartment. Angus was now a registrar. I saw him at a medical meeting not long after coming back and excitedly said hello. He looked at me without expression, looked away, and then kept walking to sit with other senior doctors. Angus didn't sit with students, he once said. From then on, he regularly delivered this kind of treatment.

Another close friend, also a registrar, said that they preferred not to have medical students around. 'I can't stand medical students,' they said before encouraging me to leave. It was just five years before then that we'd been medical students together – them even sharing tears with me.

It hurt. Most of these people used to be my friends. Now, they ignored me and talked down to me, but did a complete about-face when talking to their seniors. Then, it was all about ass-kissing. Their lips were often positioned near their consultant's booty. I swallowed my pride and kept going.

Things became much worse when I came to the surgical rotation. On the first day, I turned up to meet the team. As I was coming up in the lift, someone said hello. It wasn't a friendly hello. It was a sharp, cold hello. I looked up to see a woman who I had a turbulent relationship with in medical school. I stopped talking to her after the accident, but now she was a non-training surgical registrar. Through some misfortune, I was to be her medical student. We'll call her NTSR, or non-training surgical registrar.

Time, it seemed, had changed her more than anyone I knew. NTSR had a notorious reputation for bullying people. There were many complaints against her from all parts of the hospital. It turned out that her reputation was well-founded. She was horrible to the juniors. More than once, her interns cried during ward rounds. She not only broke people's spirits, she tried to derail their careers by mis-informing their seniors. NTSR was extra venomous to me.

One day, I was in a clinic with her. The students had their own rooms. They reviewed a patient, then went to a doctor with the story to get a final review and plan. I had a room next to NTSR. A nurse came in.

'There's a patient outside in so much pain,' she said. 'Everyone is busy. Would you mind please seeing them to try and do something about the pain?'

I said that I was only a student, but would do what I could. The patient came in and explained the problem. They had a long-standing surgical issue which that day was causing a significant amount of pain. They were visibly distressed. I reviewed the patient, then went next door to talk to NTSR.

'I don't give a f∗∗∗ about that patient, they belong to another team. You've just wasted your time,' she yelled.

The doors were open. The patient heard everything. I went back to them.

'I'm so sorry about that. There's not much I can do now,' I said.

The patient was good about it. But these incidents continued to happen with NTSR. She was awful to patients. She was even worse to junior colleagues. She called me after hours to hassle me. She mocked me. She belittled me. Every day.

I gritted my teeth and kept going. I didn't want to complain or make a fuss. There were too many eyes on me. I was just trying to get through medical school with already complex circumstances. While I got through it, the term with NTSR was easily the worst medical time of my life.

NTSR did teach me something important: humility. Eventually, her own career became derailed. She was forced to seek a career outside the hospital. The power that she wielded over people disappeared overnight. She became irrelevant to the very people she tried to dominate.

Every few weeks, I had an appointment with an academic and neurologist by the name of Tien to help with catching up academically after so many years off. He volunteered to help me get back up to speed. Tien was passionate about medicine. As a consummate physician, he knew intimate details of medicine. He challenged me. When I got things wrong, he pushed me to think more. I went away and learned whatever I messed up. I grew to appreciate his approach. It was the perfect balance of applying pressure, stimulating thought, and teaching. Through his intellectual challenges, I grew. I appreciated the importance Tien placed on under-standing the basics. I learned to love the details hidden inside medicine. Thinking back now, it wasn't so much the content that Tien taught me which was important. It was his philosophy of medicine and critical thinking.

A doctor I had on the paediatrics rotation really chal-lenged students. There were certain things that they just expected you to know perfectly. These were things like treating asthma emergencies. It was fair too, because those were conditions that could kill children quickly if not treated properly. Sometimes, students cried in the teaching sessions as a result of their style.

I had another supervisor cut from the same cloth. He used to grill me during ward rounds. If I made a mistake when presenting a patient, he cut me off abruptly. Start again. Do it again. Again. I repeated it until I got it right.

While I didn't enjoy it at the time, I've never forgotten the lessons these doctors taught me. However, I wonder how contentious these teaching methods are. While I benefited from them, some note that style to be bullying. And there's a fine line between bullying and applying meaningful pressure. But teaching isn't straightforward.

I have a medical school colleague whose previous career was in teaching. He often brings educational science into training junior doctors at work. Once, I was involved in a course by an expert educator that my medical school colleague helped to deliver. I was fascinated to learn the immense amount of science and, more importantly, art, behind teaching. The course reminded me of the Dunning–Kruger effect again – I realised that I know so little about teaching.

Teaching is a complex practice with so many nuances. In a profession where teaching is so important – indeed it is a fundamental part of what we do as doctors – I wonder if we need more formal training to be effective teachers. This is a worthwhile point to ponder, because it is senior doctors who teach junior doctors much of the craft.

And the craft is a life and death activity. That's the reality of it. Doctors are required to make life and death decisions, sometimes within seconds. The wrong decision can kill someone. So, I see the value of doing everything I can to learn to be better. I also see the value in a hierarchy, because at the end of the day someone needs to be responsible for what happens to a patient. Usually, it's the most senior doctor.

But how do we make sure that hierarchies are healthy, not toxic? One option is a 'flat hierarchy', where senior people are known and respected but approachable. In the department that I work in today, all the senior doctors are called by their first name. This is in contrast to some other areas, where the preferred way to address the senior doctor is by calling them Dr Surname. In our department, seniority can be identified by the different colours of our scrubs. While it's different in every hospital, black is the most senior in our department. This is followed by grey, then blue. The seniors in black are nearly uniformly supportive of their juniors, even regularly making sure that their personal wellbeing is intact.

In contrast, a toxic hierarchy runs on fear. If there is a problem, the junior person is less likely to approach a senior person for help. There are some departments where a consultant is never to be approached directly by anyone below the registrar level. In our department, anyone can approach a consultant with a question. Apart from the negative effect that these idiosyncrasies can have on patient care, the wellbeing of junior doctors can be affected too. We've had too many doctor suicides as a result.

When it came to study, I had a lot of cobwebs to dust off. I had been away for five years. After finishing at the hospital every day, I went to the medical school building. There, I had a height-adjustable desk that the school set up for me. High desks are great. I can lean on them with my elbows for balance. If the desk is low, it takes a lot more effort to hold myself up. Without having control of my trunk, sitting at a low desk is tricky.

At this desk, I studied for hours. In fact, I'm writing this book from the same desk, years later. I usually studied there until the last tram came, which was around 11.30 pm. Over the evening, I watched the sun set. I saw the medical school staff winding up their day. Everyone slowly filtered out. I was still there.

I read textbooks. I did practice questions. I watched videos on all sorts of medical topics. I drew things on the computer. I wrote notes. I talked to myself. I did everything that I could to learn.

Winter was tough. I tried to keep myself warm by drinking hot water and covering up with a hoodie. I tried not to move much, because then the heat escaped from my cocoon. Some nights, I shivered until I got warm again.

Professor Broadley often worked late. He was juggling two jobs as the dean and a neurologist. Some nights, it was just him and me in the medical school. On the way out, he usually stopped to say hello. My desk was right near the main entrance. Sometimes, we chatted for about half an hour. Professor Broadley told me about his experiences in medical school. He gave me bits of wisdom on how to survive. Sometimes, we just talked about life.

I don't know if he ever realised how much those moments meant to me. I often felt small after the days at the hospital. But he was someone senior making time to just talk. I felt valued. That gave me fuel to keep going for another couple of hours.

To make a difference in someone's life, we don't need to do big things. The little things count. A simple act of kindness can make an unforgettable impact. It can be as basic as a quick hello.

As the time for the last tram approached, I packed up. I knew how close the tram was getting because I had an app that kept track of it in real time. When it got just close enough, one of the trusty boys took me to the tram. If it was winter, I shivered all the way to the warmth of the tram. I was warm in the tram, then shivered again from the tram station to the house. I showered, slept for a few hours, then started the day again. I usually did this six days a week. On Sundays, I was a slob. I lay in bed, watched TV, slept, and ate pizza.

7

MEDICAL SCHOOL

Whether you think you can, or you think you can't –
you're right.

Henry Ford

EVEN IN 2021, some of the biggest Australian hospitals
were still paper based. Up till about 2015, just when I
started as a student there, Gold Coast University Hospital
was, too. When a patient came in, a pile of paperwork
needed to come from medical records. Stacks of notes,
medication charts, test reports and other documentation
were stored in stacks of folders. The doctor sorted through
the notes to figure out what had happened to the patient
previously. The notes were hard to search. The charts could
be lost. And, well, I'm sure you know how bad doctors'
handwriting can be. The whole situation created risks.
Still, our profession has been firmly attached to paper
charts for a long time.

Fax machines were also still a thing in medicine well into the 2020s. Referrals were faxed to a machine. No one knew if the paper fell on the floor and disappeared. No one knew if a random person picked the fax up to find someone's confidential health information.

The digitisation of hospitals has not only eliminated safety risks but made medicine more efficient. When a patient comes in now, most of the time, their entire history can be accessed quickly. A doctor can see their notes, vital signs, lab results and other critical information at any point in time. Sometimes, this can be lifesaving.

The best thing about digital hospitals for me is that they bridge a physical gap. If I had to mess around with paper charts without the use of my fingers, medical practice would be unnecessarily challenging. When I came back to medical school, I was thrilled to see that our hospital had just deployed an electronic medical record.

Our hospital had an abundant supply of coffee too. Coffee is the lifeblood of medicine. It keeps people awake. More importantly, it allows people to bond. A morning coffee session after a ward round brings the team together while they plan the rest of the day.

I was in the line at the coffee shop one day. Standing in front of me was the educator who had oriented us to the electronic medical record. I said hello, and she asked me how I was. Good, I said. After some small talk, I told her that it would be nice to have the electronic medical record on a tablet computer, because the computers on wheels were too cumbersome to push around while using a wheelchair. 'Let me think about it,' she said.

A short while later, the educator arranged a tablet computer with the electronic medical record for me. I could do a ward round with the tablet on my lap. I wrote notes and accessed results. This was great for the fast surgical ward rounds in particular. Suddenly, I was a more useful part of the team.

The educator who arranged the tablet for me had acknowledged a problem and solved it. There was no bureaucracy. There was no delay. There was no unnecessary complication. I was quickly made more efficient and enabled, just because someone took the initiative.

I kept figuring out ways to make myself more efficient, such as streamlining the workflow when seeing a patient, giving thought to everything from how to best write a note to the optimal direction from which to approach a bed. I also realised that most limits were perhaps only in my head. One day, I was talking to Dan Gillespie, the medical school buddy I had travelled to Japan with.

'I can reliably put a cannula into a model with a little bit of help these days,' I said.

'That's great,' Dan replied.

'It'd be cool if I could put it in a real patient.'

'Why can't you? If you can do it on a model, you can do it on a patient. It's how everyone does it.'

I didn't have a response to what he said, but the idea stewed in my head for a while. He was right.

One day, a patient on our ward needed a cannula. It was the nephrology ward where patients were notoriously difficult to cannulate due to their lengthy journeys through chronic kidney disease. *What better place to start*, I thought. I talked to my medical student buddy on the ward with me. I told her that this would be the first time I'd ever put in a cannula after the spinal cord injury, but that I'd like to try. She agreed to help.

We gathered the equipment, then went to the patient and told them the situation. They agreed to let me try. I positioned myself, prepared the equipment, and put the cannula in. Success. My buddy secured it with a dressing. I was on top of the world.

I enjoyed these victories, but still came across emotionally confronting times. The friends that I knew before the accident kept advancing in their careers. They were getting married. They had kids. Some became senior doctors in their fields. Watching them sometimes created a pang of hurt inside me. I felt left behind. I wondered if I would ever have what they did. But I took solace in the thought that we all have our own unique journey. It's rarely helpful to compare our lives to what other people are doing. It's even more unproductive to try and follow the demands of society's grinding wheel of expectations and trends.

I've had many friends who put a huge amount of value

into marriage, children, jobs, houses, money and other tick boxes equated to a successful life. They've become depressed when these things don't manifest. It's not because they actually want those things. It's because they feel like failures in the absence of achieving those things by a particular time in their lives. There's so much pressure on people to follow a plan.

The reality is, we don't need to follow a plan. It's more important for us to find our own truth and path.

It's said that Colonel Sanders, of KFC fame, could never hold down a job. He apparently had jobs in the army, on streetcars, railroads, insurance, and even as a midwife. The colonel's restlessness culminated in him inventing his special chicken recipe while running a small food outlet in a gas station. Colonel Sanders ended up travelling across the United States, trying to set up franchises. It was probably a hard life for him then. But through his efforts, Sanders eventually had over 600 franchises. The most interesting part? The colonel started his journey with KFC when he was over 60 years old.

If there's a dream, we have to chase it regardless of the status quo, social expectations or the pressures against us. We've created an idea of a socially acceptable lifestyle that has become ingrained in our psyche. It's not real, though. It's just an idea. Is a nine-to-five job really that relevant in a digital, remote-capable workplace in 2022? Why are Saturdays and Sundays the only days when one can relax? In the summer heat of Australia, what purpose do suits and ties serve? There's much in our society that we just accept to be the norm. As we move along in life, we stick to that norm more and more rigidly. With that rigidity, though, there's little room to dream.

Dreamers who change the world tend to be outliers in this very world. Think about people like Thomas Edison, Leonardo da Vinci or Abraham Lincoln. They weren't ordinary. Ordinary is following the stream, like a leaf floating on the current. Extraordinary is daring to do something different by embracing the path true to the heart, even if it means jumping out of that current. By jumping out of the current, these people eventually changed the direction of the stream.

I was thrown out of the current, violently and unexpectedly, with the car accident. I watched the people around me, floating ahead, having seemingly perfect lives. Their careers, relationships and lives seemed like things that I would never have. Much of the time, it hurt to look at the things that seemed so far from my reach. Those days, I often connected with the lyrics in the song 'It Don't Matter' by the band Rehab.

But later, I embraced the idea of walking a different path. I let go of the idea of a 'normal' life. Having shed the weighty chains of my ideas of normal, I started to see possibilities. I even started to feel free. The Japanese poet Mizuta Masahide said it best in his 17th-century haiku.

Barn's burnt down, now I can see the moon.

When I saw the moon, I realised that in my head, I once thought that the spinal cord injury meant that I was going to miss out on life. I was wrong. Disability didn't mean inability. I realised that I could have something far better than I ever imagined.

A big step for me to prove that point was still to get through medical school. To that end, I tried to make myself incrementally better every day. I tried to do the little things well. After all, big things are a collection of little things done well. A Rolls-Royce, for example, is excellent because of the sum of its parts. Every single detail has been put together perfectly.

I took this approach to medical school and life, because I knew that both of those things had to be working well for me to succeed. From the way I kept the house to the way I wrote study notes, I tried to do everything well. I knew that if I didn't do the little things well, I couldn't do the big things well. There are many who liked this idea, such as poet Emily Dickinson who said, 'If you take care of the small things, the big things take care of themselves.' And Fernand Point, the father of modern French cuisine, who said, 'Success is the sum of a lot of small things done correctly.'

Small things matter. I had a study buddy in medical school who used to get incredibly frustrated with me. When we studied together for the practical exams, I used one of a million mnemonics to remind myself to wash my hands, gain consent from the patient, explain what I was going to do, invite questions, prepare equipment if necessary, have appropriate lighting, expose the area of interest adequately, and position the patient in the right way. Simple but important things. I did this for every practice session with my buddy, over and over again. If I cognitively offloaded these simple things into a mindless routine, they were easy marks to get in an exam, and I could concentrate on the more complex tasks. My buddy hated it, because they said that such minutiae is not necessary to repeat constantly. But then, my buddy very nearly had to repeat both of the final years.

Similarly, I streamlined life. Emails got attended to once a day, in the morning. Bills were automatically deducted from my credit card. The clothes were washed and ironed in a certain routine. The wheelchair had a daily checklist. All the mindless things offloaded to run smoothly so I could pay attention to the big things.

Eventually, the first set of exams approached. I told everyone that I wouldn't pass them because I'd been away for five years. It would probably take me time to get back into the swing of things, I said. While I said that outwardly, inside of course, I wanted to pass the exams. I wanted to do well. Underpromise and overdeliver. I wanted to prove everyone wrong. I kept studying as hard as I could. Even the windows in my room were full of medical scribbles written in marker pen.

The exams came. I finished the main written one in about half the allocated time. I checked it over several times, thinking that I messed up. I went to the bathroom at least six times, which is how I discovered that nerves make me pee a lot.

I passed.

From that point on, even more people started to believe that I could do it. The number of disbelievers kept shrinking. Even I started to feel more confident. *This can work*, I told myself.

There is much unseen work that goes into a result. Michael Jordan said that he missed thousands of baskets, but we only saw the ones he sunk on TV. Edison said that he discovered thousands of ways not to make a light bulb. Graeme Clark, the inventor of the bionic ear, sacrificed everything to help people hear again. Socialising, indulgence, sleep, comfort and security are often traded for a dream. That's what I did too. I barely ever went out to socialise. I didn't sleep much. I was often uncomfortable, whether it was the cold, fatigue, pain, fear or emotionally confronting moments. The work and sacrifice that goes into a result is never as visible as the result itself. In my case, it was the same.

Our medical school had a student who kept failing. They failed repeatedly for many years. They had one final shot at passing before facing exclusion. The student, who was junior to me, reached out to ask if I would study with them. Of course, I said yes. I made time to go through some material with them one night. But as I tried to review it with them, it became apparent that they weren't interested in the material at all.

'What tricks did you use to get through exams?' they said.

'Well, I can tell you some strategies I used to learn things.'

'No, I mean, how did you get around the system?'

'I just spent a lot of time studying.'

'What I'm trying to ask is, how did you talk them into letting you pass?'

This student thought that I had used some underhanded methods to pass. They eventually went to staff at the medical school to quiz them about the same thing. What shortcuts did I take to pass? Was I afforded some special deal? This student thought that having a spinal cord injury precluded me from passing on merit alone. They failed again, and were excluded. I've come across attitudes like this once or twice since then. I've brushed them off and kept going.

The further I got into medical school, the more I realised how much I loved it. Apart from the patients, the intellectual challenges of medicine gave me much satisfaction.

During one medical term, I had a consultant who was old-school. He taught by challenging people publicly. On a ward round once, we came across a patient who was ill with sepsis and low blood pressure, but also had severe heart failure. The situation was dire.

'What would you do for this patient now?' he asked me.

'I would give him a lot of fluids to bring the blood pressure up.'

'You may have just killed the patient. They have heart failure. They won't be able to pump the fluid around. Why did you choose that?'

'It's what the guideline for treating sepsis says.'

'Your job as a doctor is to think. The guideline might tell you one thing, but your job is to critically analyse situations. That's why you get paid.'

I never forgot this lesson. He was right. The world is protocol driven. In medicine or elsewhere, there's often a guideline to follow, but it may not really contain the solution you need.

This is a frustration even in our day-to-day lives. How many times do we come across the bureaucrat on the phone working step by step through a script? There's little room to move. There's no room for heart. Our world is sometimes so risk-averse that we forget the human at the other end. We need to always remember to be flexible when helping people. In those situations, only morality matters. Not the rules on paper. Most importantly, the rules shouldn't stop us from exercising common sense.

This consultant was an interesting character. He was of the opinion that for a doctor to be taken seriously, they must drive a nice car. He drove a prestigious, expensive car. Hierarchy was important to him. He was often short with the staff, and regularly with patients, too. He was the guy who told a patient that all their problems were caused by their weight before storming off – 'it's because you're fat'.

Having said that, I learned a lot of medicine from this doctor. You take the good from people and leave the bad. There's always something to learn. He also highlights the dichotomy between technical skills and human skills. They are sometimes mutually exclusive. Like this consultant, some have one but not the other. I think that in any vocational pursuit, the two should be married.

In medicine, for example, it's not enough to just have human skills. There's no point being nice to your patient if you don't know how to save their life. At the same time, there's no point in expertly managing someone's diabetes if you're going to destroy their soul in the process.

I was running on the hope that I wasn't too much of a dick to patients or colleagues. So, I kept working on my technical knowledge.

My friend Ben and his now wife Laura regularly set aside time to help me study in those days. Ben was the one who dealt with all that aftermath from my accident. They lived in a different city by this point and had a little boy, Charlie. They were both working as busy registrars. Nevertheless, they made time to call me once or twice a week. We sat on the phone and went through various medical topics. Ben talked to me about general medicine, his specialty. Laura talked to me about obstetrics and gynaecology, her speciality. They took it in turns to teach, then quiz me.

To this day, I try to pass on that kindness to other medical students. They did it for me. I do it for others. Kindness is like a torch that way. We have a responsibility to keep passing it around.

It's also said that you can easily judge the character of a person by how they treat someone who can do nothing for them in return. I could do nothing for Ben or Laura then, yet they treated me well. I think that speaks volumes about their character.

While my journey through medical school was ticking along, other things were happening in my life. Over time, I had to deal with health issues. Weight gain was one. I managed to put on about 20 kilograms in the first year back at medical school. A large part of it was my diet. A rehabilitation physician told me that with a spinal cord injury, there aren't many sensory indulgences. Taste is one of the only senses remaining. Because of that, food becomes one of the few sensory experiences one has. And you know what, it's true. Tasty food is one thing that I can still feel.

On top of that, most of the muscles in the body aren't being used anymore. The calorie requirement is much less. For a man with my characteristics without a spinal cord injury, the calorie intake might be somewhere around 2500 to 3000 calories per day depending on their level of activity. For me, it's about 1600 calories per day. To put that into context, a Big Mac has 563 calories. A slice of white bread might have around 66 calories. To go through an entire day without blowing out the calorie count takes discipline. If we are putting in more energy than we are using, then the excess energy input gets stored as fat.

I got annoyed with buying progressively bigger pants. The breaking point was when I was told that I needed a new wheelchair to fit my newfound bulk. I started counting calories on a phone app. After militaristically sticking to the calorie restriction, I dropped about 22 kilograms in six months. This meant, however, that I lost some helpful padding on my booty. The subsequent pressure caused a tricky wound that took some time to resolve. Everything is a fine balance.

Sleep also became problematic. Weight gain contributes to poor sleep. But also, respiratory muscles don't work properly in people with spinal cord injuries. When you fall asleep, your airways can collapse easily. That's sleep apnoea. When this happens, you wake up, sometimes without even knowing it, because the body becomes short of oxygen. When I did a sleep study, we found that I was waking imperceptibly multiple times an hour. It was no wonder I was often – am often – tired. To this day, we haven't been able to solve the sleep problem properly, even with a machine that helps me to breathe at night.

Pain can be another complex part of a spinal cord injury. Some people suffer from severe pain caused by the broken nerve endings firing off abnormally. I often get chest pain. It's been investigated thoroughly and put down to pain from the spinal cord injury. It doesn't bother me much anymore, but it's often there.

By then, despite all these little challenges, I fortunately had enough reasons to keep going. Our reasons for living matter, because they make the obstacles in our way smaller. Indeed, Friedrich Nietzsche said, 'He who has a why to live for can bear almost any how.'

8

THE POWER OF ONE,
THE POWER OF MANY

When bad men combine, the good must associate;
else they will fall one by one, an unpitied sacrifice in a
contemptible struggle.

Edmund Burke

IN MEDICAL SCHOOL, there's sometimes an opportunity to
spend some time in an area of interest within or outside your
home school. In Australia, this is called an elective. Before
the accident, I always dreamed of doing an elective at the
Harvard Medical School. Harvard regularly ranks as the top
medical school in the world. It's also the oldest in the United
States. It has a rich history full of medical discoveries and
amazing people.

After the accident, I didn't think that this would be
possible anymore. How was I going to travel to an unfamiliar
foreign country? I'd never been to the United States before.

I had no idea what it was like for someone with a disability there. I didn't know what it would be like to fly for around twenty hours. It was so far from the safe zone I had built.

I talked to Mum about my thoughts one day. She said, 'Why not?' She told me to just do it. The worst thing that could happen is that we get on a plane, then need to come back.

So, I applied to spend some time at the Harvard Medical School. I told them about my spinal cord injury. They didn't care. They offered me a spot in radiology. I was to be the first ever visiting medical student with quadriplegia to their knowledge. Mum and I set about planning how to spend a couple of months in Boston through the thick of winter.

We looked around for accessible apartments and found one right next door to the TD Garden arena where the Boston Celtics play. We booked our air tickets. The day quickly came around, and Mum and I flew to Los Angeles, then New York. It was snowing when we finally arrived in New York. The drive in our road transfer to Boston took about four hours. Those hours went quickly, because there was a lot to look at outside the window. The snow was incredible. When we got to Boston at about 2 am, we settled into our apartment and shared a pizza before falling asleep.

I've been to the United States a couple more times since then. It turns out that I've been flagged as a security risk for some reason. On my boarding pass for any American-bound flight, 'SSSS' appears. This means that I have to go through a rigorous security check. I'm usually taken into a room, questioned, searched, then released. I'm not sure what kind of terrorist they think I am, but the process is as entertaining as it is tedious.

Flying for that long isn't fun when you have a spinal cord injury. My legs move around everywhere. There's little balance for the trunk when the seat is upright. It's cramped. The occasions when I've been able to wangle my way into business class have been bliss.

Flying can be deadly for someone with a disability. In 2021, a disability activist ended up dying in the United States after complications resulting from the airline damaging their wheelchair. Really, getting around in general can be problematic. Once, I parked my car near a café to have coffee with a friend. I put the disability parking permit on the dashboard. After a little while, my friend said, 'Someone is fiddling with your car.' I looked around. Someone was letting down my tyres. He was a shabby-looking middle-aged guy dressed in jeans and a black hoodie. My friend and I wandered over.

'What are you doing?' we asked.

'You don't have a parking permit.'

'Look on the dash,' I said.

It then turned into a scuffle and the guy ran away. This wasn't uncommon. More than once, people have approached me while I'm parking in an accessible spot – sometimes yelling.

Scuffles with parking vigilantes aside, in Boston, I was attached to the Massachusetts General Hospital, the number one ranked hospital in the United States at the time. Founded in 1811, the hospital boasts achievements like the first public demonstration of anaesthesia and the first successful replantation of a traumatically amputated limb. As of 2021, thirteen Nobel Prize laureates came from the hospital.

Winter was cold in Boston. I once left a glass of water on the balcony to see how quickly it froze. It didn't take long. For me, who couldn't control my body temperature, it was a taste of hell. Well, a very cold hell. But I had a strategy. Every morning, I turned up the heat in my room to the max. I used hot packs. I overheated my body to the point of discomfort. Then, when I went outside to the snow, the cold was refreshing. I often wandered to the hospital in just scrubs. By the time I got there, my body had cooled down to a near-normal temperature. Bostonians were usually kind-hearted. Many thought that I was homeless during my wander to the hospital and offered me blankets or jackets. When I did get there, some would say, 'Man, Aussies are tough.' I was okay with both these misunderstandings, especially when attractive American women offered me their jackets.

In the hospital, I set about learning as much as I could. The radiology clerkship, as they called it, was very structured compared to my time elsewhere. There were daily teaching sessions and clinical time. I spent as much time in the hospital as possible.

It was a true academic environment. If I had an interest in a particular topic, there was always someone willing to teach it. All I had to do was reach out to that expert. Curiosity was rewarded. The doctors I came across were happy to teach. This is not always the case elsewhere, like some parts of Australia, where hospitals are purely operational. North American doctors often compare their system with Australia's in noting that in the US, junior doctors are considered people primarily in training. Delivering clinical care is a secondary priority. In Australia, junior doctors are said to be first and foremost people involved in service delivery. Training is a secondary objective, often done in their own time. Training is important. We could probably use a bit more emphasis on that in Australia.

Until that point, I had only read about what was happening in the spinal cord injury research world. In fact, I read many scientific papers talking about advances in spinal cord injury research with much hope. I saw my time in America as an opportunity to connect with spinal cord injury researchers in New York and Boston. I emailed a few. All of them agreed to meet me. One notable example was Professor Yang Teng, known as Ted. Ted was a thoroughly respected spinal cord researcher leading the way globally.

Ted later told me that he looked me up online before agreeing to meet me. Luckily, my online footprint must have been okay, with the leaked nudes from university safely hidden in an invisible corner of the web. We met at his lab in Harvard. It looked like a proper science factory. There was unique-looking machinery, experiments in progress, and the odd student.

We made our way to his office. Ted asked me about my background and I told him a little about my life. Then, we launched into talking about spinal cord injuries. We spoke about some of the science forming the frontier of spinal cord injury recovery, as well as everything from stem cells to drug therapy to electrical stimulation with promising applications in treating spinal cord injuries. Ted was a next-level intellectual. He explained some of the biological mechanisms that might lead to spinal cord injury therapies and treatments. It was arguably the most intellectually stimulating conversation I've ever had. When our long talk finished hours later, Ted and I agreed to keep in touch. I left his lab with my mind buzzing, energised and excited.

I think we undervalue how much there is to gain from having conversations with new people. I once met Jesse's great-uncle Adrian over lunch. Uncle Adrian was in the top 10 tennis players globally in the over-90s age category. He had spent a bit of time in Ethiopia as a diplomat. One day, he was invited to the office of Emperor Haile Selassie. Apparently, the Emperor had a lion in his office. People were terrified of the animal. I wonder if the lion was kept there partly as a tactic to unsettle visitors. Whatever the case,

Uncle Adrian decided that the lion would be tame from sitting in the office all his life. So, as soon as he walked into the office, Uncle Adrian approached the lion to pat him. As expected, the lion was tame. Impressed by Uncle Adrian's courage, the Emperor ended up becoming lifelong friends with him.

There's a lot to take away from that story, but I wouldn't have heard it had I not taken the time to listen to this man who had a lifetime's worth of knowledge and experiences to share. Conversations are important.

In between medical school commitments, Mum and I looked around Boston. We watched the Celtics play. We ate gluten-free cannoli, because I wanted to see what all the fuss from *The Godfather* was about. I tried a bison steak. We also made a trip to New York one day. There, we went up to the top of the Empire State Building. It was night-time. The city looked magical from there.

The time flew by. I finished my term at Harvard, earning a distinction with honours. It was the highest attainable grade. The first visiting quadriplegic medical student at Harvard had done his stint, and now it was time to come back to Australia.

I launched into my last year of medical school. More exams came, and I passed. For the clinical exams, the school engaged an external independent observer. The idea was to independently verify that I was performing well, that everything was above board. I wanted them there. I wanted to show the world that I had earned this. The observer agreed that I performed well.

About a third of the way into that final year, the time came to apply for a job. In Australia, all domestic medical graduates are guaranteed jobs. What's more, I had a scholarship with the state health department which included a contract to work for them through five years as a doctor. When applying for jobs, applicants rank their preferred hospitals. A ballot system then sorts them into their final positions. I applied like everyone else. But there was one difference. I disclosed my spinal cord injury.

Not long afterwards, I received a letter stating that my application had been removed because of the spinal cord injury. There was to be a 'bespoke process' to consider my circumstances. Initially, a short timeline was provided for this process, although there was no detail about what it would involve. Time started to stretch. Months went by. I provided medical assessments; I provided letters of support. More months passed. I still had no idea what was happening with the mysterious process. Meanwhile, my colleagues had received their jobs.

At the end of the year, I passed all the exams. I was eligible to graduate as Queensland's first quadriplegic medical graduate. Sarva flew in from Sri Lanka for the graduation. I still remember the smells, sights and sounds from that time. I just discovered the song 'Old Thing Back' by The Notorious BIG and it was a staple. Sarva, Dilith and Varuni gifted me a blue Paul Smith suit and shoes to wear for the big day.

I graduated with awards. Professor Broadley spoke about how he hadn't been sure whether this moment would be possible, but was glad that it was. He said that it was one of the best moments of his career. He acknowledged my mum with a gift of flowers on the stage. I gifted him a broad-sword. As I later came across the stage to get my degree, the entire hall celebrated. For me, Mum and our new family from the medical school, this was one of the best moments of our lives. There was nothing but happiness. I was elated. At one point, this had all been a dream. In that moment, the dream became reality.

The media covered the graduation, and they asked me whether I had a job. I still didn't. They turned up the heat on the health department.

In December, I was registered as a doctor by the Medical Board of Australia. The health department then incorrectly told the media that the delay in finding me a job was because I had no registration. At one point, it was said that I was the only domestic medical graduate in Queensland without a job. I particularly enjoyed the headline, 'No job as top doc sits and waits'.

I had the opportunity to attend a political event with some prominent politicians in power around that time.

They gave speeches about equality, fairness and justice. That's what they stood for, the politicians said proudly. There I was, listening to this speech while being denied employment because of a disability with no deficiency in merit. The air was thick with hypocrisy. I was angry.

While the health department dithered, I reached out to some other states. New South Wales and Victoria agreed to have conversations with me about pursuing jobs in their jurisdictions. However, it had to be a year later because all their jobs were then taken. The Australian Capital Territory said that I wouldn't be treated any differently from a graduating doctor without a disability. They put me on a waiting list for a job because their positions, too, were filled.

I spoke to some of my legal colleagues. They connected me with John Sneddon, a prominent lawyer who had won awards for civil justice. He was involved in notable cases, for example freeing political prisoners trapped in foreign countries. He cared.

We talked about the potential for success if this became a legal matter. It would've been a challenging fight. The same department had once won a case against a nurse who had a mild traumatic brain injury. The nurse had difficulty working night shifts due to some symptoms, but had no cognitive or motor problems. The nurse asked to be excused from night shifts. The department said no. The case eventually reached one of the superior courts, where the nurse lost her appeal with costs.

That was the state of affairs. Instead of finding a way for an injured nurse to gain fulfilment in a vocation while contributing to the economy, the department decided to punish them. How many resources would have been expended in that unjust endeavour? The bureaucracy can be heartless and often without common sense.

Health staff who acquire disabilities or illnesses are forced to go through tedious return-to-work processes, often to the detriment of their wellbeing. Another doctor who acquired a spinal cord injury was told that he couldn't work in his hospital, because the wheelchair would be a safety risk. 'What if you fall off?' they asked. How ironic it is to make such a case in a place that uses so many wheelchairs for its patients. Another senior staff member was asked to work from home because they were using crutches due to a foot fracture. Apparently, the crutches were deemed to be a safety risk. Again, the irony. Hospitals have huge stocks of≈crutches that we hand out to patients daily.

All this happened while the department website boasted of being an inclusive employer that doesn't discriminate based on disability.

I was frustrated. I didn't know what I would do for an income the following year. Mum and I invested everything in the medical school journey, and now I was at the end of it with no job.

Someone from the department told me that I wouldn't be starting work with my colleagues the following year.

Another spokesperson from the department forbade the Gold Coast University Hospital from communicating with me. That person directed me to communicate with them and them only. They didn't offer me a job, but they did offer free access to their mental health service because they felt that I would be distressed. I wasn't distressed. I was even more annoyed.

I was fortunate to have the support of the media, community, doctors, academics, politicians and just plain old good people who believed in doing the right thing. There's power in grassroots movements. Institutions, governments and establishments are accountable to the people. Think about movements like Black Lives Matter or Me Too. Institutions bent to the voice of the people then.

At the end of the day, these institutions respond to public pressure. If it's going to affect votes, share prices, sales and such things, institutions will respond to those calling for change. For example, a social media campaign once asked consumers not to buy Danone-branded products in Morocco, protesting against the company's high prices. Danone's Morocco-based subsidiary lost 40 per cent in sales and suffered a big loss as a result. Private institutions care about money.

Outside of activism by the people, the media is an important check and balance in a democracy. Thomas Jefferson said, 'The only security of all is in a free press.' Napoleon said, 'Four hostile newspapers are more to be feared than a thousand bayonets.'

Institutions, too, are susceptible to public opinion because it will eventually affect someone's vote. Many politicians care very much about votes. A politician once told me, 'The only thing that matters in this game is numbers.'

So, the numbers matter. The people have power to move those numbers. I think it's often underestimated how much power people have if they care enough. I, too, had some luck thanks to people who cared.

By this time, I had spent a lot of time in the emergency department at our hospital. Growing from the seed Lauren initially planted, I felt at home there. I liked what they did. I liked their culture. The emergency department was like a family. They looked after each other. Lauren wrote a letter of support for me to get a job. Some of the emergency physicians offered up parts of their salaries to fund my job. Many people asked questions. Politicians wrote letters. The media did more stories. A community supported me. It worked.

On the Friday afternoon preceding the Monday when the baby doctors were supposed to start their jobs, I was having a beer with a friend. We were talking about what I was going to do that year. We were tossing around jobs that I could take to keep myself afloat. During that conversation, I got a phone call.

'I'm calling from the Gold Coast University Hospital,' the voice said. 'We would like to offer you a job, starting on Monday.'

9

THE DOCTOR WILL
SEE YOU NOW

Impossible is just a big word thrown around by small
men who find it easier to live in the world they've been
given than to explore the power they have to change it.
Impossible is not a fact. It's an opinion. Impossible is
not a declaration.

Mohammad Ali

I HAD NO cash reserves when I started as a doctor. I used
my credit card to buy some business clothes and shoes,
and spent that Saturday and Sunday feverishly preparing
to start work on Monday. My mind was so prepared to be
unemployed that the idea of starting work took a bit of
getting used to.

I was due in the hospital early on Monday. I woke up
at the usual ungodly hour to get ready. This day, I wasn't
catching a tram as a student, but as a doctor.

I arrived at the hospital for orientation. It was scary. Starting work as a doctor is scary for anyone; the idea of having someone's life in your hands, even under strict supervision as a baby doctor, is nothing to be sneezed at. Doing that with quadriplegia just amplifies the nerves.

The media came to cover my first day. They asked me how I felt. 'Excited, but terrified!' was my answer. Some of the journalists had taken the whole journey with me, so we were all happy to see that day come to fruition.

We spent two weeks in orientation, which covered things like prescribing, referrals, ward rounds and other basic topics that the medical intern should be able to do. There were also the tick-box exercises mandated by human resources. Some of these were pointless online activities, often to mitigate a risk that has appeared on a bureaucrat's radar at some point. No one learned anything, but the organisation can say that their staff was trained in whatever topic it was – usually at a significant cost.

An example of this type of reactivity was seen during COVID-19. A key part of the personal protective equipment were N95 masks. These masks were effective at keeping out the virus. However, they had to be fitted properly. That required fit-testing each individual. All this was well-known before the pandemic.

During the pandemic, a Queensland hospital experienced some failures in personal protective equipment. Subsequently, the nursing union held the health department to account. It was said that N95 masks were not being fit-tested for staff. Suddenly, the department mandated that all staff in all hospitals had to be fit-tested. The testing measurements had to be recorded. This happened within a tight timeline. Every day, we received emails asking us to get fit-tested. It didn't matter if staff worked in areas with no COVID-19 patients. Fit-testing was mandatory. They wanted it done rapidly.

This is reactivity. It's risk mitigation subsequent to an adverse legal event. If there was a focus on quality and heartfelt care for staff, fit-testing would have happened early in a controlled manner.

Many mandated training modules for healthcare staff often come from a reaction to something. Often, there is nothing meaningful to gain from it apart from the organisation being able to discharge their responsibility. For medical staff, these modules are generally done in our own time outside of work.

I also had to complete training that other doctors didn't need to do. I sat in a room for the better part of a day learning about occupational violence and its management. The hospital thought that I was at higher risk of experiencing violence.

The hospital and I then planned how I was going to tackle the year. The medical intern has provisional registration as a doctor. To gain full registration, they have to fulfil certain requirements during that year. This includes successfully completing several rotations in certain specialties. A key question for me was which medical specialties to do. That involved a conversation with a doctor who looked after the interns.

He was a good man, but an occasionally intimidating one. It wasn't unusual to see him storming around the hospital yelling profanities about subpar management by other doctors. Still, he had a heart of gold. We set up a meeting. He said to me, 'We need to do this year in a way that is not tokenistic, not too easy, and has credibility.' There are some specialties well known for having less than vigorous workloads. I was not to spend too much time in those specialties. We decided on psychiatry; obstetrics and gynae-cology; vascular surgery; general medicine; and extended time in emergency medicine. Vascular surgery in particular was known to be a spirited specialty. But I was going to be starting in psychiatry. Just as in student life, it had a better pace for me to get used to being a doctor. In contrast to being a student, though, I had actual responsibility now.

During my time in psychiatry, I was still figuring out how to do some things. As an intern, many tasks were new to me. But sometimes the problems came from unexpected quarters. I had a colleague who was just barely my senior on our team. From very early on, they stopped talking to me. If I said good morning, there was no reply. They often didn't share the patient list with me. They didn't discuss what was happening with our patients. Most of our interactions were filled with awkward silences, with them not responding to anything I said. I still have no idea what that was about. I must have got them offside at some point. I loved the work, but dealing with this colleague every day wasn't fun. I tried to ignore it and keep going. I just needed to get through the internship. To my relief, the psychiatry term quickly came to an end.

Everything is a big step in early intern life – even prescribing paracetamol. What if I cause liver failure? What if the patient has a reaction? When I had days off, I was terrified that I would come back to find that some monumental error had killed someone.

This is not far-fetched. Remember the grumpy doctor who drove the prestigious car? In a moment of vulnerability, he once told us about losing a young patient to a pulmonary embolism. This is a blood clot that gets lodged in the lungs. It can be fatal. Ever since he lost the patient, that doctor has been extra vigilant about pulmonary emboli. Medicine does that. When we make an error, we swing far the other way to being overcautious, sometimes to the point of detriment.

My colleagues have experienced the sudden loss of paediatric patients, adult patients, and even people they have known personally. The marks left by these losses are deep. Imagine carrying the death of someone with you.

As an intern, you learn more about the medical hierarchy. The medical student is more insulated because they have little responsibility. The intern is responsible for things, and they answer to those above them. Those above aren't always forgiving. Ryan Holiday said in his book *Ego is the Enemy* that, 'It is a timeless fact of life that the up-and-coming must endure the abuses of the entrenched.' In medicine, the entrenched wield power not just by virtue of seniority, but by the influence they have on a junior's career. They can make or break it.

There are also power differentials between specialties. Radiology, for example, is at the end of the line. Everyone needs something from them, but radiologists rarely need anything from anyone else. Therefore, requests to radiologists can be met by snappy rebukes. Emergency medicine refers patients to every specialty. Other specialties, apart from general practice, rarely refer to emergency medicine. This creates a power imbalance that sometimes results in difficult conversations. The way people behave in situations of perceived power differentials sometimes shows the dark side of the human nature.

Hospitals are therefore a unique social microcosm. In a 1963 article called 'The Social Structure of a General Hospital', Robert Wilson says, 'Because its work goes on around the clock and its life-sustaining goals demand a maximum of self-sufficiency, the hospital constitutes an internally diverse society within a society.'

To me, since I was a student, the emergency department was always a good society fostered by great leadership. They employed a flat hierarchy. Consultants were happy to be called by their first names. This created an environment in which an intern could approach the consultant without fear. In some other specialties, the unspoken rule for an intern is never to contact the consultant directly. I've seen a breach of that rule result in retribution affecting a person's entire intern year.

Even though the emergency physicians were great to their interns, the interns couldn't be shielded from the harshness of other specialties. One night, for example, I was sitting next to another intern in the emergency department. It was late; approaching midnight. An ambulance accidentally delivered a terminally ill young cancer patient who was actually intended for a private hospital to our emergency department, and the intern assumed care of them. The patient was normally looked after in that private hospital, who had all their records. The staff there were familiar with them and knew what this patient needed to be comfortable. The family hoped to arrange the prompt transfer of this young patient to the private hospital so they could be somewhere peaceful and familiar, away from the chaos of an emergency department.

The intern called the private hospital. The nursing staff there were happy to accept the patient. However, the on-call oncologist needed to accept the transfer. Those were the rules. So, the intern called the on-call oncologist. Nearly immediately, I heard their screaming response over the phone.

'I don't give a f*** about this patient. They belong to another oncologist. Don't ever f***ing do this again,' they shrieked, and continued with a long tirade full of expletives. They refused the transfer.

The intern cried. They finished the shift, then cried some more in the car park. The patient stayed in our emergency department till the morning, until another on-call oncologist started at the private hospital. This type of thing is sadly too common in medicine.

In Robert Wilson's 1963 article, which still remains relevant today, he said, 'Unfortunately, the patient is often the battleground of professional competition; his body, mind, and purse are scarred by the zealous attempts to do for him what each staff member's specialty dictates. The hospital, too, is a battleground often ripped by a crossfire of professional purposes.'

Medicine isn't easy. Aside from the weird social structure within, the technical demands of the job are high. Mistakes can kill people. Chaos can ensue within seconds. We are thrown into complex situations regularly, without warning. Training is long and arduous.

While medicine is criticised for these things, I think there is some basis for the way it is structured. The hierarchy is necessary, because at the end of the day someone needs to be responsible for the patient. If there is an adverse event, the responsibility often falls on the person at the top of the food chain. Why wasn't the surgeon adequately supervising their junior? Why didn't they double-check the order? Most problems become the responsibility of the senior-most doctor.

Training needs to be long and arduous, because at the end of the journey you are going to be that senior-most person. People will look to you for a decision. You will be responsible for everything, including the lives of multiple patients simultaneously.

For all its complexities, though, I love being a doctor. The opportunity to be challenged, to learn every day, to grow, and to do all that while helping someone is a unique privilege. Medicine humbles me daily. It teaches me to be a better person, much through my interactions with the humanity within it.

Later on, when I was doing the intern term in general medicine, administrative tasks were common. Many of the general medicine patients had complex social issues. They didn't fit neatly into another specialty like cardiology. Therefore, there was a lot more going on than medicine alone. It was easy to get caught up in the mundane tasks of the day, forgetting why we were there – the patient.

One day, I was leaving work after a long day in general medicine. It was early evening. I was tired. Just as I exited the ward, a nurse ran after me.

'Are you finishing up?' the nurse asked.

'Yeah, I'm just leaving.'

'That's okay then. The family of that terminally ill patient just wanted to talk to a doctor. I can get the ward call doctor.'

I knew that the ward call doctor wouldn't know this patient. At night, the ward call person looks after a large number of patients. They often tend to minor tasks like recharting medications. They don't assume the ideal continuity of care for a patient like this.

I stopped at the door for a minute. I had a choice. I was off the clock; I could leave and forget about the whole incident. Or, I could go back and talk to the family about where we were at. I had the ability to explain everything clearly as a doctor from the treating team. I knew that the family would benefit from a chat with a doctor familiar with the patient. I went back. The family were grateful.

That moment at the door allowed me to reflect on something that I haven't forgotten to this day. For me, that was just another day at work with many patients. For that family, it was one of the biggest events that they'll go through in their entire lives. We're faced with these choices all the time. Do we decide to be a human or a drone?

When I rotated into the vascular surgery department, the days became much longer. Ward rounds started anywhere from 6.30 am to 7.30 am. For me, that meant waking up between 3 and 4 am.

Preparing the ward round is the junior-most doctor's job. The ward round is based on a list comprising all the patients under a team's care. There may be patients who have been around for several days. Others may have been admitted overnight. The list should generally contain basic demographic information about the patient, their primary issue, other problems, relevant clinical information like lab results, and a plan. Before the ward round starts, the responsible doctor should create or update the list, then print copies for the team. The team then moves around the ward, seeing each patient on the list, while making a plan for the next steps. The junior-most doctors create a task list for themselves during the round, which is to be completed through the day. The task list might include things like arranging referrals, organising scans, or discharging the patient.

Here, I tried to use whatever resources I had as a strength. Remember the tablet the educator in the coffee line organised for me? It had remote access to the hospital's medical record. I wanted to take the load off my other junior colleagues, so I arranged the list every morning while having breakfast at home. When we got to work, the list was ready for the team.

Aside from work on the ward, vascular surgery had clinics and operating theatre lists. I wasn't often in the operating theatre, giving my eager colleagues more of an opportunity to experience it. Instead, I attended to the other jobs. There was enough work to go around for the whole day.

The vascular surgery team liked to have an evening ward round too. There were three junior doctors on our team, so we took turns staying back on alternate days. Some days, I didn't get home till 9 or 10 pm.

As long as the days were, we had a blast. Regular but short post-ward round coffee sessions gave us time to get to know each other. Every now and again, we had dinner together. We had tough days, but we got through them together.

At the end of my time in vascular surgery, I sat down with a senior surgeon for my review. He said that I had excelled. He concluded by saying, 'When I first heard that you were coming to work with us, I was unsure. I didn't know what to think. Today, I'm disappointed in myself for thinking that way. My perception of what medicine can be has changed.'

We are quick to make judgements. It takes humility to allow the evolution of those judgements. Sometimes, this never happens. Sometimes, it happens, making room for respect.

After graduating as an intern, I obtained full registration and became a resident. I was even a nominee for an intern of the year award. I started plotting out my career plan in earnest.

Early on as a junior doctor, I met two specialists to talk about a prospective career in a certain specialty. The first was supportive, and congratulated me on getting so far in my career. They spoke to me alone first, then called a second specialist. I'll call the second one Palpatine. This doctor was a key decision-maker in who would be accepted into specialty training at the hospital. They wielded this power over potential trainees, sometimes making them jump through many hoops just to be told that they're not good enough.

Without even saying hello, they immediately became aggressive. 'I have so many concerns about you coming to this specialty. Can you even type?' they said. I could. I learned how to type at about sixty words per minute with my knuckles. After a period of telling me about why I couldn't do one of the less physical specialties in medicine, Palpatine ended the conversation.

Some specialties in medicine require you to be liked by the entrenched people within the system. In this one, too, it's an unspoken rule that potential trainees meet all the key specialists at various hospitals. Those doctors size up the trainee, then give feedback about their prospects of entering the training program. Many specialists, both inside and outside my hospital, were supportive of me, but by no means all.

Over the subsequent period, I felt that Palpatine was taking it upon themselves to derail any career aspirations I had in their specialty. One attempt was to tell me that they wouldn't pay me to work in their department. They asked me to find my own salary to work, whether it be as a resident or registrar. Then, I understand they asked the hospital for extra money to have me as a junior doctor for a term.

When I worked for them as a resident, I felt that life was complicated. I felt I was at Palpatine's mercy. As the junior-most doctor, I was at the bottom of the pecking order for certain tools required to work in that specialty. Often, the tools that were accessible to me were taken. When I asked about finding these tools, Palpatine's answer was that I should 'take them from a consultant'. By this point, you will know that I could never ask a consultant that.

Research was another important aspect of building a career in that specialty. I was involved in two research projects during my term. I stayed late nearly every day and collected data from hundreds of patients for a couple of weeks. I wrote a notable amount of the draft paper for that study. Palpatine apparently asked other team members to exclude my name from the studies, then to present them without giving me any credit.

One day, I emailed Palpatine to ask for their reasoning for their approach to me. Instead of replying to my email, they sent me a text message asking me to call. When I did so, they said, 'You just can't work in this department. We can't have someone with a spinal cord injury here. I don't want you to tell anyone that I said that. If anyone asks, you need to tell them that it's the position of our entire department that you are not wanted here.'

This dislike of me was probably amplified by some of the politics within that specialty. I wondered if I had friendships with specialists who were disliked by the leadership. Some of them hated each other. It wasn't unusual for a consultant to feverishly criticise another in a public space, in their absence. The specialty had enemies outside itself too. It has in the past come under public scrutiny for their practices.

For example, you know those pesky mandatory modules? Well, Palpatine once asked the residents to go around and do them all for the consultants and registrars.

Palpatine then sent another specialist to have a conversation with me. 'The politics mean that you can never work here in the future,' they said after pulling me aside one day when I happened to bump into them. At another event, the director of junior doctors called me over. They said that a discussion with the department had taken place. 'You should consider a career outside clinical medicine. Leave those things to people who have the physical capacity to do it,' they said.

I had a contemporaneous record of all these events. I even had some emails. When I summarised it all to a human resources director, their response was essentially, 'Move to a specialty that's supportive.' The union for doctors was powerless. No one could do anything.

Having someone attack you based on physical differences is heartbreaking. That's why racism is so destructive. Discrimination based on physical ability is just as destructive. It strikes at the core of your being, because the attacks are focused on attributes over which you have no control.

Having said that, there's no point allowing someone's bigotry to dictate your life. Anger can destroy us. I once read a story about a python that found a knife. It initially wrapped itself around the knife. As the knife caused it more pain, the python became angrier. It wrapped itself tighter around the knife. As the pain increased, the python tightened their grip even more. Eventually, the knife killed the python. Anger is like that. If we hold on too tight, it destroys us from within. It's one of the ways in which the Palpatine of *Star Wars* created Darth Vader in the series. And hey, I don't want to become Darth Vader.

According to Buddhism, pain arises from our attachment to things, and attachment to hurt causes more pain. The only way to relieve the pain is to remove attachment from past hurts.

I once had a girlfriend who was bullied in high school, where she had been an outcast, the uncool kid. She carried this hurt into her adult life. She often made comments like, 'I bet you prefer that preppy rich girl who plays tennis.' She hated her mum because of things that happened while she was growing up. She didn't trust men, because her dad had left. She had insight into all these things. She explained it all to me. But she was never freed from the hurt. I felt for her. I often wondered, though, how long can you go on letting those feelings dictate and destroy your life?

I tried to take responsibility for my feelings so that I could move on from events that caused hurt, like Palpatine's behaviour. I don't hate them. I forgive them. And that is liberating.

Apart from my rotations in psychiatry and that specialty, the rest of my terms as a junior doctor were filled with good times. In my intern year and second year, I spent time in obstetrics and gynaecology. I must like unpredictability, because obstetrics and gynaecology is loaded with it. There are some incredibly special moments, like when a baby is born. I've been in the room when new life comes into the world. I've even been sprayed with amniotic fluid. Apart from the magic of the moment itself, it always made me think back on the journey that my mum must have taken.

The special moments can quickly turn, though, when things go terribly wrong. Mums can start bleeding critically. Babies can get sick inside the womb. Time is of the essence. There's no room for mistakes.

The obstetrics and gynaecology juniors had some busy days on occasion. One Christmas, I was the only resident floating around for some reason. I had three phones. That day, I counted at least fifty phone calls. One of them was from the ward about a complication from a Bakri balloon. This is a device that can be inflated inside the uterus if a mother is experiencing ongoing bleeding after delivering a baby. It stops the bleeding by applying pressure. I arrived at the patient's bedside. I had no idea what to do. I called the registrar, but she was in the operating theatre. There was no one else around to help. A theatre nurse put the phone to the registrar's ear so she could talk to me while operating.

'Get down there and tell me what you see,' the registrar said.

I got down in between this patient's legs and described what I saw.

'Okay, you need to pull it out,' she said.

She gave me some brief instructions and hung up the phone. I called her back. I had never even heard of a Bakri balloon before, let alone seen one. Neither had the nurse looking after the patient. It was an intimidating prospect to pull something I'd never seen before out of someone's vagina. The registrar reiterated that it was a simple task, and directed me again to pull it out. To be absolutely sure, I looked up the details again online, and they matched up with the registrar's instructions. The nurse and I pulled it out. For the record, the patient was okay.

The obstetricians and gynaecologists were supportive of me. The midwives were excellent. I once delivered a baby with a midwife, Lauren Skinner. The baby's mum took a photo with us. A couple of years later, the mum returned to have her second baby. She was with Lauren again and fondly remembered our time together at her first birth. These are the moments that make medicine special. Lauren and I have been friends ever since I was a student.

I learned about medical storytelling too. Medicine, like advertising, likes a good story – but that story has to be delivered quickly. These are stories delivered from doctor to doctor when they are discussing the clinical care of a patient. Medical students generally go into too much detail. Without clearly delivering important points, they'll go through the history, examination, investigations, and on occasion the diagnosis with the plan. The intern will quickly refine this technique, because they soon realise that they won't last long if they're not able to tell a compelling story quickly. The senior doctors are veterans at getting the story across fast. In general, the story should take 10 to 20 seconds for an uncomplicated patient. If it takes longer, you can sometimes see the senior doctor's attention wander. Their eyes will literally dart away. Some will ask you to move on. Some will interrupt.

I remember calling an anaesthetist once to tell them about a stroke patient who was going to the operating theatre for a procedure called a clot retrieval. In this procedure, the blood clot in the patient's brain is retrieved using a minimally invasive method to restore blood flow.

'I just wanted to let you know about a stroke patient coming up to you for a clot retrieval. They have a history of –' I started.

'Stop there,' the anaesthetist interrupted. 'So, a stable patient is coming up for a clot retrieval?'

'Yes.'

And they hung up.

It's not that doctors' attention spans are short – they just want to know the important information in a timely manner. Apart from ensuring a focus on the vital information, saving time is also important. Say there are 40 patients to be handed over to the morning doctors from the night ones. If each patient took four minutes, the handover would take 160 minutes. That's nearly three hours. If each patient took three minutes, that's still two hours. That's a significant delay for the morning team to attend to patients. Stories need to be brief while getting the critical details across. Storytelling in medicine is a skill that takes time to develop.

Apart from the time limitations, the patient handover is important for safety. Handovers are associated with errors, the most serious resulting in death. It's said to be the most common root cause of adverse events. The World Health Organization prioritises handovers as a major safety issue. Handovers are described as the point where 'safety fails first'.

Communicating quickly and effectively is important not just in medicine, but anywhere. I learned this first in the business world. People's interest needs to be snagged quickly with a compelling argument. This principle has grounding in some real-world evidence. A 2015 study of 2000 Canadians by Microsoft found that a person's average attention span was about eight seconds. We have eight seconds to grab each other's attention.

Communication was important in every single specialty I tried. As I moved along with my medical career, I learned the nuances of what different specialists want to know about their patients. Over the first couple of junior years, though, I kept coming back to the emergency department. It felt like home. Eventually, I started working there constantly without rotating to other specialties.

10

A QUADRIPLEGIC EMERGENCY DEPARTMENT DOCTOR

I would like to see the day when somebody would be appointed surgeon somewhere who had no hands, for the operative part is the least part of the work.

Harvey Cushing

Medicine in places like emergency departments, general practices and rural areas is unpredictable. One minute, you might get a critically ill trauma patient on the verge of death. The next minute, it'll be someone with chest pain leading to a new diagnosis of cancer. Then it'll be someone with a sexually transmitted illness. Next might be a stubbed toe. You see a rich tapestry of human existence and experience a broad continuum of emotion.

I like to think that frontline medicine is a window into our society at any given time. It's something of a thermometer for the extremes of what people are going through. Crime, drug abuse, trauma, domestic violence, chronic disease, homelessness, pandemics – or whatever it may be – frontline doctors see the fluctuations within the community many times a day.

Around 2020, our emergency department was the busiest in Australia. We were seeing more than 100,000 patients annually. A notable proportion of these patients had psychiatric illnesses. Some were suicidal. Some had psychosis. Some were depressed. Christmas was variable. Mondays were usually busy. 'Quiet' was a taboo word which, if inadvertently uttered, would cause all hell to break loose. Holidays dedicated to the defence forces brought back memories in veterans, who then came to us in distress.

With some of these conditions, the patients are brought in involuntarily. Emergency services have the power to present the patient for assessment if there was a risk to them or others. The time limit for assessment was 12 hours. However, this can be extended for a period of time through other paperwork. Coming from a lawyer's view, I'm fascinated by how easily someone's liberty can be taken away from them. Sometimes, a staff member will come to a doctor requesting that a patient be made involuntary. The doctor may not even have reviewed the patient, but staff will still sometimes push the doctor to facilitate an involuntary order to contain a patient. It's an act that is fraught with risk.

Our mental health services were under such siege sometimes that I might finish my shift in the emergency department and come back the following day to find a patient still waiting to be assessed by someone in psychiatry. In some hospitals, the environment for awaiting assessment is prison-like. They are bare rooms with only a mattress and stainless-steel sink. Imagine that. You are going through depression, thinking about ending your life. Then, you end up alone in one of these rooms involuntarily for over 24 hours.

Domestic violence presentations are commonplace too. Sometimes, it was sickening. We had patients arrive in the department who were unrecognisable due to the violence inflicted upon them. We had patients who escaped after having been kept prisoner and repeatedly assaulted in the most hideous ways. Then, there were the subtle cases. The wealthy wife who says she fell but the injury patterns don't match. Their medical history demonstrates a concerning string of injuries. You dig deep; the truth comes out.

People with disabilities experience domestic violence more than the general population. Some data suggests that women with disabilities may be about 37 per cent more at risk of domestic violence than their peers. Men are affected too. And I can see how it happens from my own experience.

I once dated a woman who we'll call Shona. When we first met, she was kind. There was a gentleness about her that everyone around her noticed. The first couple of months were good. One day, I was at her place when I noticed a voicemail on my phone. It was from a female friend. I played it in front of Shona; I had nothing to hide.

'Hi! I haven't seen you for so long. I miss you. Call me back!' my friend said.

Suddenly, Shona turned. The look on her face was one I'd never seen before, a mixture of anger and hesitation.

'What the f*** was that?' she said.

'That's my friend,' I explained.

Shona became uncontrollably furious. She smashed her fist against things around the house. 'Men are so f***ed!' she screamed. I was shocked at the whole outburst. She thought that I was cheating. This behaviour continued for a couple of hours, at which point I gave up trying to explain that the voicemail was from a friend. I left.

The behaviour kept escalating as time went on. We were once at a crowded park. Shona thought that I checked out a woman who I hadn't even noticed. She screamed and ran away. At its peak, there were episodes like this every couple of days. She became jealous of any female friends or colleagues. She asked me to cut them off. Shona started going through my phone without permission, looking for evidence of infidelity. She went through my emails. I had female friends, but my social life was an open book. And what's more, I would never even think about cheating.

Shona insisted that if I moved in with her, she would feel more secure. I suspected that this was a means of control.

I knew that it would be a disaster, so I kept saying no. We tried counselling, but she wouldn't stick with it. The counsellor encouraged her to see someone on her own, but she didn't.

It turned out she had a history of being violent to partners, where police had been involved. Slowly, even more concerning behaviours started to emerge. Shona threw a phone at me once. She pushed me without warning, and I nearly fell. Both times, she laughed and said, 'Oh now you're going to hold that against me.' I wasn't scared of her, but the red flags made it clear that a long-term relationship would never work. Even her mum pleaded with me to end the relationship for the sake of my safety. After trying for a while, I ended it.

The point is, it's easy for anyone to slip into these relationships. Even I did. Too many don't make it out. In the emergency department, I've seen people die at the hands of their violent partners.

Relationships are complicated. When I was travelling in Japan with Dan, I read the Gabriel García Márquez book *Love in the Time of Cholera* while on a night train. It's a book about the complexities of love in Colombia through the late 1800s into the early 1900s. Well, I can tell you, love in the time of a spinal cord injury is even more complicated.

My physical self is different now. I'm comfortable in my skin. I love my life. But it doesn't offer a normal relationship to someone. The intimacy is different. Shona once said, 'I don't feel close to you because you can't be physical with me like normal.' Even though she was an unusual character, I sometimes pondered the idea. Should I deny someone those normal things? Would it be selfish to pull someone into my unusual life?

I ended up staying single for a cumulative total of about 10 years after the accident. I was like a monk, though a happy one, focused on work. Maybe that's why monks make great beer and wine – they are able to have a singular focus on it, unfettered by their desires. In those 10 years I rarely felt any human touch resembling intimacy. I didn't realise that until many years later, when a woman touched my hand during a normal friendly interaction at work. I hadn't felt anyone's touch that way for so long. Although purely platonic, it felt electric. I don't feel much of my body these days, so the parts that I can feel are sensitive. I soaked up the magnitude of that moment. Human touch is a wonderful thing.

Still, I found myself avoiding relationships for a long time.

Having said that, there are people of all abilities that do relationships well. The wheelchair tennis star Dylan Alcott's relationship with the sexologist Chantelle Otten was notable for its success, with Chantelle famously saying that it was the most amazing thing. Stephen Hawking, Christopher Reeve and Nick Vujicic all had great relationships, too.

Okay, maybe I just liked being a bachelor.

I also wanted to look after my mum. She's given up her own marriage, career and aspirations to get me where I am. She's made sacrifices. I owe her everything. If I were to be in a relationship, the other person would need to understand the role that my mum plays in my life.

A lack of relationships, and its by-product, loneliness, does get to people. It's been the reason for suicidal thoughts in many patients I've seen, particularly in the elderly. Even though we are more electronically connected than ever, we are disconnected as people. A large part of the time, social media isn't about helping people connect. It allows us to view the seemingly perfect veneer of someone's life, which can create doubts in us about our own. All it takes is a chink in our mental armour for these doubts to seep in and consume us. One day, we wake up to find ourselves chasing a picture-perfect moment that didn't really exist for anyone except the camera lens. It's damaging, especially to the fragile persona of youth who are still developing into fully fledged humans.

In this environment, connection is so important. That's why sometimes the biggest impact we can make in medicine is by just talking to patients. There is no technical skill, no procedure and no drug that will do this for us. It's just about sharing some time as two human beings.

I remember a mum who nearly lost their child to significant trauma. It was approaching midnight. The mum was distraught. A nurse came to get me to see if I could help.

There really wasn't much I could do, but we found a corner where she could have a seat. I got her a cup of tea. We talked.

'I get it. My mum was where you are right now a few years ago,' I told this mum.

'Really?'

'Yes. I was critically injured. She was so distressed.'

We talked for a bit longer. The mum became calmer. She wasn't okay, but felt a little better. She went back to the intensive care unit to be with her child. Much later, she wrote about this experience online. Our chat had apparently made a big difference that night. I had no idea that our conversation had helped so much, but I'm glad it did.

It's rarely our technical skills that really create a lasting memory in people. I don't think that my Bakri balloon patient will remember me for expertly pulling out the device from her vagina. I don't think that the heart attack patient remembers that I gave them 300 milligrams of aspirin. I don't think that the patient with belly pain remembers that one of the tests I ordered was a lipase. Hopefully, they just remember that I cared. Hopefully, they felt safe.

Our technical skills become second nature. But human skills are easily forgotten.

The spinal cord injury gave me the opportunity to connect even better with other patients like me. One busy night, the department was full. Staff were running around everywhere. Ambulances waited to offload streams of patients. Even at about 2 am, we were a hive of activity. An ambulance delivered a patient who had a genetic condition which affected the formation of bones. The patient was prone to fractures because the bones were brittle. The patient used a wheelchair. I was to be their doctor that night.

'As soon as I saw you come up to my bedside, I knew that you would understand what I was going through. I was happy,' the patient said.

This was one of the most memorable moments in my career. To that patient, my spinal cord injury was an asset.

Despite all this, it might be apparent to you now that doctors with disabilities haven't always been welcome in medicine.

Shortly after I came back to medical school, the deans of medical schools in Australia and New Zealand created a policy that sought to exclude students with disabilities. I found out about their intentions early on in the process after I became privy to an email distributed by one of the committee members who drafted that policy. A part of the email said that the guidelines 'do not bind us to exclude anybody but it is hoped that they will provide some legal protection where we do have to make the difficult decision that a candidate's disability cannot reasonably be accommodated to enable them to study medicine'. I knew the person who wrote that. It felt like a stab in the heart.

They wanted legal protection to enable the exclusion of medical students with disabilities. If those guidelines were applied to me, I could easily have been excluded. The guidelines included things like motor function, sensory function and the ability to understand social cues. How many doctors have you met who are dismissively socially inept?

Over the years, there was a great deal of advocacy to change these guidelines. Various reasons were given to maintain them as they were. Some were responses like, 'What if we get a tsunami of people with disabilities who want to be doctors?'

Being a doctor is primarily a cognitive activity. Physicality is no longer the primary need for many areas of medicine. Numerous doctors don't perform CPR, because there are other people in the hospital who do that. In 2022, we even have machines that can perform CPR and assist with procedures. I've played with a robot that can drive a wire into someone's brain to deploy a stent. I can easily work the controls with no finger function.

In 2020, the medical deans finally started redrafting the guidelines. A year later, an inclusive set of guidelines was released. This time, instead of being called inherent requirements, the document was titled 'Inclusive Medical Education: Guidance on medical program applicants and students with a disability'. Driven by a passionate team, the document aimed to promote inclusion with statements like, 'Proactive promotion of inclusivity is also an approach – for example, assessing the accessibility of learning environments against universal design principles.' In a few short years, inclusive medical education came a long way.

I still wonder, why try to exclude people with disabilities in the first place?

I know many doctors around the world that practice with disabilities. There's a quadriplegic emergency physician, a paraplegic surgeon – a few actually – and even a blind physician. Despite these trailblazers, I still came across barriers years into my career as a doctor.

I once had an informal discussion with the Australasian College of Emergency Medicine about training in that specialty. Not long afterwards, I received a letter in response without any warning. The letter said that the college would not accept an application from me to train as a specialist in their program, although they would consider other pathways. It was topped off with a patronising sentence, 'Please note that the decision outlined above in no way detracts from the admiration that the College or its individual members or staff have for you and your achievements in the profession of medicine to this time.' When I subsequently had a meeting to clarify their position, I got nowhere. The final letter noted that I was being antagonistic, as I was asking questions preceding it.

Despite the college's poor attitude, I have had many emergency physicians who supported my career. I remember having a chat with Dr Stuart Watkins after that period with the college. He said, 'The more senior you become in your career, this matters more than those.' He pointed to my head, then my hands. 'I work with you. I know how you are as a doctor. A piece of paper doesn't matter to me.' Stuart spent much time teaching me how to use the ultrasound in the emergency department to expand my skill set. Another doctor, Dr Charles Britton, spent months with me figuring out how to do various procedures so I could earn a different qualification in emergency medicine.

Like them, there were other great attitudes too. When I talked to the Royal Australian and New Zealand College of Radiologists, they found a way for me to work around the procedural aspects requiring fine motor skills in their specialist training program. After all, I wouldn't be performing those procedures anyway. In their view, I just needed to understand how and when those procedures would be performed.

Equally, the Australian College of Rural and Remote Medicine was brilliant, with some of their specialists even inviting me to train in their program when I met them at a conference. The rural doctors told me that they liked a challenge and opportunities to think outside the box.

In the end, I realised that all these interactions were the best things that happened to me. Not only did they expose the variety of attitudes within medicine, but helped me find where I belong best.

While we were advocating for changes in the policies locally, the conversation for inclusive medicine heated up globally. I had the opportunity to provide some written

support for a court case for medical students with disabilities in India. I participated in an American campaign
encouraging medical students with disabilities and gave
input to similar work in the United Kingdom. I also got the
opportunity to travel to San Francisco to speak at Stanford
University at a conference called Stanford Medicine X.
Initially, I thought about speaking at the conference remotely
to avoid the tyranny of flying, but Mum encouraged me to
go in person. It was one of the best things I ever did.

Mum and I took the long flight from Brisbane to San
Francisco. San Francisco was beautiful, and Stanford was
amazing. I presented my talk, which covered my journey
then made some points about why inclusion in medicine
is important. There, I met author Jeremy Howick, who
wrote a well-known book titled *Doctor You*. Jeremy and I
immediately hit it off.

Over the next couple of years, Jeremy kept encouraging
me to write a book. He encouraged me to reach out to other
authors who have published books in Australia. On Jeremy's
advice, I connected with the Australian author Jamila Rizvi.
Jamila is a seasoned author who knew exactly how to help
me publish a book, so she too took me under her wing. The
rest is history. Here I am, writing the book – all because
Mum encouraged me to take a trip to Stanford, where I
talked about disability and medicine. My life has been full
of sliding doors moments like that.

I also spoke at TEDx in Brisbane about being a doctor

with a disability. TED is unique. The organisers strictly curate the content of your presentation. They arrange an initial meeting to vet you. Then, they begin to craft the speech with you. I wrote the initial draft, which was about 3000 words. The TED team edited the whole thing. There was a certain way they wanted sentences to be structured. The speech needed a specific tone: the TED tone.

Once we refined the speech, it was time to memorise it. Yes. They wanted me to memorise the whole speech word for word. There weren't to be any departures from the wording written in the draft. I had to deliver it by memory with specific intonations.

The actual event was attended by about 700 people. Apparently, thousands more watched live online. It was the single most nerve-racking talk I have ever given, simply because of the pressure to perform. It was also one of the best learning experiences I've had in public speaking.

The message for inclusion in medicine spread even more. Change started to happen in Australia, with policies, guidelines and position statements encouraging inclusivity. Apart from the medical deans bringing out a new guideline, the Australian Medical Association in Queensland spearheaded a position statement which became a national position. It laid down the importance of inclusion within the profession. Many conferences began to include topics on inclusion within medicine. Some specialist groups developed special interests in inclusion. Internationally and nationally, people reached out to me about inclusion. At the same time, there was an impact on other professions, in the health sphere and beyond.

As the environment for doctors with disabilities saw a rapid change in the world outside, I was enjoying my time in the emergency department.

To make timing easier, I started working mostly evening and night shifts thanks to rostering by my bosses. The evening shift started at 1 pm and the night shift at 10 pm. These shifts made the wake-up time for my little family much easier. The 4 am starts for the 7.30 am day shift weren't the easiest for my team.

Night shifts brought their own challenges. There are generally no consultants in the hospital through the night. If you need one, they are about twenty minutes away. Therefore, the registrars are in charge.

One night, all the registrars were tied up in simultaneous resuscitations. It was about 2 am. Some of the patients needed to be intubated – that is, have a tube inserted down their throat to help them breathe. These kinds of patients are usually very ill. They need a lot of human resources.

I was a junior resident dealing with some other patients. One had a drug overdose. Another had sepsis. A third had diabetic ketoacidosis, or DKA. This is a complication of type 1 diabetes which can be life-threatening. It can be a labour-intensive condition to manage. All three of my patients were getting sicker by the minute. I was juggling those three while managing bits and pieces for other patients in the department. Because the registrars were busy, the interns were coming to me with questions.

There are times in medicine when you just don't know how to get through the next few hours because of the workload. I mean, I've actually stopped a few times over the years and thought, *I have no idea how I'm going to get through this*. But you have no choice. You just have to keep going. This is also probably nothing compared to what, say, rural doctors experience in their demanding jobs.

It's a great feeling to get through these pressure-cooker moments. When coming out the other end, you've grown. Next time, you handle it better. I've grown to enjoy these shifts.

As fun as the pressure can be, it's an emotional roller-coaster too. More than once, I've made a new diagnosis of cancer for patients around my age or much younger in the middle of the night. Some of these patients had kids. Some were just barely out of childhood. While it's sad to find a diagnosis like that in anyone, these patients made me think about my own mortality.

I was grateful for these moments, because they reminded me to go home and appreciate the people I love. They also reminded me to keep living as much as possible.

What does living actually mean? I have a friend who pursued a career as a life coach. Their job was to teach people how to live well. In their coaching, my friend equated good living with a series of rigid rules. This, according to them, is the road to happiness. You must sleep eight hours between 9 pm and 5 am. You must never eat anything other than organic food. You mustn't use electronic devices.

Some of this isn't too far off the truth. Eating more fruit and vegetables is great for your health. Sleep performs functions that will help you live a long life. Electronic devices can be pathologically addictive. In my humble opinion, though, a good life isn't so formulaic. More importantly, there are people who feel that they fail at living well if they don't stick to these formulae. It's damaging.

I'll sleep a little bit less if it means that I can spend more time with a loved one. Every now and again, I'll eat a pizza. I use electronic devices to entertain myself when I like.

Apparently, Margaret Thatcher slept around four hours a night while Mariah Carey likes to get about fifteen hours. Warren Buffett loves Coca-Cola and burgers. The Rock likes video games. Regardless of our opinion of them, these are all people who have made an impact on society. Everyone is different. And that's okay. As long as we find happiness in our own unique way, that's all okay.

In my journey to find happiness, I learned to seize opportunities too. I know that tomorrow is not a given. I want to make the most of today, at least for now. Like Richard Branson, I'll 'say yes and figure out how to do it later'.

I think that this is particularly important in the early

career. You can't afford to say no to things. When I was a medical student and junior doctor, I said yes to everything. Opportunities were like nuggets of gold, because I was not only a junior but someone with a spinal cord injury. I wanted to grab every chance to become better. I said yes to every research project that came my way, which eventually made a mark on my CV. I said yes to the presentation at Stanford, where I met amazing people. I said yes to helping streamline processes, which improved the efficiency of hospitals. There were nights when I went through thousands of medical records one by one, recording how the patient was managed so we could improve care. I didn't count the clock. I never bothered about the paycheque. I learned a lot. Doors opened. I'm better for it.

Years after my accident, I met the trauma surgeon who fixed my spine. He had a reputation for excellence. He was always seeking to make things better. It was in his blood. With regards to work ethic, though, he once said that we share the philosophy of 'doing extreme work'. That is, working to take something to an extreme end. I suppose what he meant is doing something like climbing Mount Everest or running an ultramarathon – all examples of extreme work. He said that one way to find excellence is to do extreme work, then work backwards from there. If you've climbed Mount Everest, then the hill down the street will be easy to climb well. If you ran the ultramarathon, it's much easier to run one kilometre well. He said that my journey was an example of extreme work, and that now I could work backwards from it.

But you know what, we need to create a society where anyone can do their work. A politician once told me that society should reward effort, but also that we have a responsibility to create an equitable playing field for anyone to make that effort.

Over time, my medical career opened my eyes to how lucky I am to be health-literate. I was able to navigate my way through a few of my own health issues which would have been difficult to diagnose had I not been a doctor.

The mild autonomic dysreflexia had been a sign of underlying problems in the summer of 2019, when I started sweating on the left side. My shirts got soaked, but only on the left. There was a perfect line down the middle. My left arm would be dripping with sweat. The left side of my face was often beaded with it.

I learned that if I have pain on one side of my body, the dysreflexia can cause profuse sweating on the other side. So that time, I knew there must be something wrong with the right side of my body. I spent a bit more time figuring out what made the sweating worse. When I lay down, it resolved. When I was sitting, the sweating got worse. This meant that there must be pain from an area that was aggravated when I was sitting up.

I tried to be a patient rather than a doctor, so I took this information to my GP. 'You're probably sweating because it's summer,' he said. I tried to explain the issue, but quickly realised the futility of my efforts. I went to work the next day. I was sweating so profusely that I frequently had to wipe the desk down.

Dr Lauren Stephenson happened to be the boss that day. I talked to her about what was happening. She pulled me off the floor, assigned a doctor to see me, and we got a CT scan. The scan showed a problem right next to the bone near my right booty. I underwent a procedure to alleviate the problem and after treatment, the autonomic dysreflexia stopped.

In the same way, we once found a fracture on my right foot. A doctor in the community didn't listen. Luckily, I again had a good boss who listened to what was happening.

This is one of the reasons I'm lucky to be a doctor. I've been able to navigate these health issues with some expertise. Sadly, most people with disabilities don't have access to the knowledge or resources that I do. I often wonder how many serious issues are missed, particularly in the developing world where access is even more limited. Globally, people with disabilities are at a higher risk of nearly all negative outcomes, including premature death. This issue really reared its head during the COVID-19 pandemic.

11

THE BUTTERFLY EFFECT

We are members of one great body, planted by nature.

Seneca

LIFE WAS ZOOMING along really well for me. Then, in late 2019, it all changed. Not just my life, but the whole world.

We started hearing rumours about a new virus that had sprung up in China. There was little information, but it was said to be a respiratory virus that potentially had some bad effects on the lungs. I wasn't worried. After all, we had SARS and MERS, which had promptly disappeared without affecting us much in Australia. Like them, the new virus was said to be from the coronavirus family.

The virus had made the leap from an animal to a human. I would love to have observed that moment when a viral particle floated from the animal to that person: that one moment that changed the world forever. Imagine that.

That person would have had no idea that this single transfer of viral material would kill millions of people.

We probably won't ever know who that person was. At one point, it was said to be a 55-year-old man from the Hubei province. Who knows for sure? He would have gone home that day. A few days later, he might have developed some symptoms. He probably thought that it was a cold or flu. The virus might have jumped from him to two or three other people. Although estimates varied, at the time this was said to be about how many people one person would infect in an uncontrolled environment. Three might have become nine. Nine might have become 27. Twenty-seven might have become 81. It wouldn't be long before over 100,000 people were infected. Those people started flying around the world. When people fly, they spend hours and hours in an enclosed space. They share air and surfaces. When the plane lands, hundreds of people potentially carrying the virus are released into another country.

It's a hell of a butterfly effect.

The first confirmed case of COVID-19 in Australia turned up in Melbourne on 25 January 2020. The first case in Queensland was in March 2020. That person ended up in our hospital.

The reality of the situation started to become clear. The virus was spreading worldwide. It was in Australia now too, spreading more and more. Elsewhere, people were starting to die.

I wandered into the doctors' common room one after-noon. There was a group of doctors standing around a computer. They were looking at a CT scan of the chest. It looked horrible: the lung fields were obliterated by infection. The tube from a ventilator was visible in the throat. I remember thinking it'd be a miracle if this patient survived.

'Whose CT is that?' I said.

'It's a COVID-19 patient,' I was told.

We all looked at the scan silently for a while. No one said anything. I knew that all of our minds were trying to process the spectre that loomed so close.

Right down the corridor from the doctors' common room was the designated COVID-19 ward. Going past it was eerie. Outside was a COVID-19 cleaning trolley. I remember looking at it and thinking, wow. COVID-19 could be living on this trolley right in front of me.

In the medical world, academic discussions about COVID-19 were all the rage. Journals started publishing a range of papers. Most provided free access to COVID-19 articles. The sheer volume of articles around COVID-19 was paradoxically unhelpful. It created a lot of noise, which made it difficult for doctors to separate useful information from junk. There were over 100,000 scientific articles about COVID-19 published in 2020. Many were peer-reviewed too quickly. Some high-profile papers were retracted.

We got excited about therapies like hydroxychloroquine and remdesivir. Some countries started to stockpile these drugs. It was reported that some Australian billionaires bought millions of doses of hydroxychloroquine. Leaders around the world touted these drugs as the solution. Many were not. The more important problem was, there were other patients relying on these drugs to manage diseases like rheumatoid arthritis and lupus.

One of the senior doctors in our hospital was drinking plenty of tonic water. Tonic water contains quinine, which is related to hydroxychloroquine. 'The evidence is weak for hydroxychloroquine, but it's not going to hurt,' he said. I guess he was right. He wasn't the only leader who was on the edge.

One of the hospital chiefs ran into me in a corridor once. 'This will be a disaster,' they said. They told me that they thought we would run out of intensive care beds. They said, 'We'll inevitably be overrun by patients. We'll have to choose who lives and dies.'

I learned something about leadership that day. It's a risk to scare the troops, to appear fearful. Like a virus itself, fear can be contagious. Fear was spreading through our ranks.

This fear was a particular problem for some staff who were from overseas. One evening, I was working in the emergency department with a colleague. Her home country had been hit particularly hard by the virus, nearly to the point of being overwhelmed. Her family was there. She was visibly distressed. At one point through the night, she was staring blankly into space. I observed her for a few minutes, then said hello.

'Are you okay?' I said.

'No. I'm terrified about what will happen to my family back home.'

We drove home together that night so she didn't have to go alone.

A doctor friend in another city rang me one day. He had a medical condition which made him more vulnerable to the effects of the virus. 'I'm getting the f*** out of this city. Everything is going to be f***ed. I'm going to go hide in the country,' he said. The fear was clear in his voice. He asked me if I was escaping too. I was not. I didn't want to leave at a time when we were needed the most.

Our hospital set about preparing for the worst. There were high-level meetings happening all the time. A command centre used in emergency situations was activated. It was staffed by the senior-most people in the hospital. In liaison with the state, they were going to run the show.

The air was thick with anxiety. You could feel it when walking into the hospital. Everyone seemed on edge. Not many people were smiling, if any. We had a program that managed bullying in the workplace. Reports to the program were at an all-time high. People were at each other's throats. A part of the reason for that was simply idle hands. Idle hands truly are the devil's playthings, because they can cause people to fight. The hospital was not busy. Everyone was staying away. There was no trauma because everyone was at home. For once, we were over-resourced.

Even though the hospital wasn't under pressure, staff were stressed. The fear remained. This was a stressful job already, but that baseline level of stress had been elevated. Some of our staff started to experience emotional challenges. Both in Australia and overseas, we began to lose colleagues to suicide. Overseas, we lost colleagues to the disease itself.

Every time we had a sniffle, or even the hint of one, a COVID-19 test was required. From memory, I ended up having five or six tests over a few months.

As the virus gained a foothold in Australia, restrictions began to tighten. Cafés closed, except for no-contact pick-up options. Traffic disappeared. Non-essential outings were restricted. It all happened quickly.

Viruses depend on some close contact to spread. If there is no spread, the virus dies within the host or sadly sometimes with the host. Therefore, physical distancing and lockdowns work in the right circumstances. They're not easy, but they work. The virus dies a natural death without new hosts to infect. However, this has a huge economic effect.

The businesses in our neighbourhood suffered. We knew the café owners. They were devastated. Some faced the loss of their businesses. To support them, Mum bought coffee and meals from them every day. But nevertheless, their losses mounted.

While the economic effect was significant, the notable ancient Roman Cicero once said that the health of the people is the supreme law: *Salus populi suprema lex*. Roman statesmen reportedly said that you must have a healthy population for the economy to thrive. If your population is ill – or worse, dead – the economy takes a big hit.

The spinal cord injury potentially put me at an increased risk of death from COVID-19. My lung function is only a fraction of what it was before the injury. The virus could have potentially overwhelmed my lungs quickly if I caught it. Working in a hospital increased the risk of transmission, but it was a risk that I was willing to take. I didn't want to shirk my duty. This is a risk that I discussed with Mum, who gave me her blessing to keep working. We agreed to have an elaborate routine when I got home, so that I wouldn't bring the virus into our house.

These kinds of routines were common among staff. One of my colleagues had a child with an autoimmune condition. He was staying in a different house while working. Others had converted their garages into decontamination zones. They had elaborate processes to clean themselves there before entering the house. And hey, I drank a heap of tonic water too.

This was a time when healthcare workers were considered heroes. In one of his talks, the emergency physician

Cliff Reid defines a hero as someone who does the right thing in difficult circumstances while weathering risk in order to help others, without the expectation of personal gain, and often while overcoming fear. A hero has a strong moral compass. They persist despite setbacks. If we go by this definition, the pandemic was a time of heroes. So many around the world rose to that standard.

It wasn't just healthcare heroes. We saw leaders around the world initiate lockdowns to protect the populace, despite protests that may have ensured their political demise in the next election. Difficult decisions had to be made. It was the police, fire fighters, paramedics, postal workers, and everyone who stayed inside. People stayed away from their families and jobs to the detriment of their wellbeing, to protect the community.

Although many celebrated them as heroes, healthcare workers faced some detractors, too. Some of our staff were spat at in the community. Some were told to stay away from public places, because of the thought that healthcare workers could be carrying COVID-19 on them.

A person working for one of the big Australian banks lived with a junior doctor during the early pandemic. The bank manager was aware of these living arrangements. They asked their employee to choose: either stop coming to work or tell the doctor to move out. The two housemates had to find alternative living arrangements for fear of the bank employee losing their job.

Some of my own caregivers worked with others in the community.' They had clients who asked them to stop working with me in case I spread COVID-19 to them.

It was a frightening time for people with disabilities, because at the start of the pandemic, we began to face serious social threats around the world. In the United States, human rights bodies started to field complaints about healthcare rationing. The *New York Times* reported that some healthcare providers were exploring the possibility of deprioritising people with disabilities from accessing life-saving therapies. People without disabilities were prioritised over them.

The National Institute for Health and Care Excellence in the United Kingdom published a critical care guideline in response to the pandemic. For frail patients, people with long-term physical or intellectual disabilities and the elderly, a different pathway was available. One could potentially justify referring these patients to end-of-life care or denying them intensive care based on the pathway. There were arguments that this was just a guide, but then why did it exist at all? At the very least it implied that less care could be justified for people with disabilities.

This conversation opens up an ethical rabbit hole. Nonetheless, there are a couple of schools of thought that are worth considering. The Maximin principle seeks to maximise the welfare of those at the lowest level of society, thus creating equity. Some utilitarians argue that this could be a waste of resources and that only those with the highest chance of surviving should be given the resources.

If you had me, a thirty-six-year-old with a spinal cord injury and poor lung function competing for a ventilator with a thirty-six-year-old without a spinal cord injury, who would you give the ventilator to? It's a loaded question. Don't worry. I wouldn't make you decide. I'd ask you to give it to the other guy. But this is not what I would want for anyone else with a disability.

Luckily, the Australian and New Zealand Intensive Care Society said that where patients are otherwise similarly ranked in clinical priority, access to intensive care must not be based on discriminatory considerations like gender, sexual orientation, disability, social status or race. They went on to say that if situation arises where patients are similarly ranked in terms of clinical priority, some legitimate instances where it may be ethically justifiable to consider other determinants for prioritisation include support for patients belonging to groups subjected to social disadvantage as a means of redressing their vulnerability and to consider that adults with caring responsibilities be prioritised.

I'm proud that Australia took a different approach from the rest of the world, both by preventing the pandemic from overwhelming the nation – at least for a period of time – while trying to protect the rights of those who are vulnerable. This involved a significant amount of national discourse. I had the opportunity to appear before the Disability Royal Commission on the topic. The Royal Commission was to investigate violence, abuse, neglect and exploitation of people with disability. At the highest level of national enquiry, we dissected the healthcare risks that people with disabilities faced during the pandemic.

I also had the opportunity to appear in the media. The most notable of these appearances was on the show *Q&A*, which fields panellists with an interest in a particular topic. Due to travel restrictions, I joined from a remote studio. It was difficult to hear the rest of the panel through the earpiece, but I tried to add something meaningful. I aimed to talk about how people with disability are at higher risk of death, and of experiencing healthcare rationing – deprioritisation in healthcare – as well as other things like the difficulties we face accessing services during lockdowns. I don't remember how much of this I got out.

One of my bosses says that the ratio of ears to mouth also reflects how you should use them. That is, listen twice as much as you speak. I don't know how well this works on national TV, though, particularly remotely. Still, all these conversations helped guide our nation in the right direction.

Intensive care requirements for a COVID-19 patient were significant. They needed to be turned in bed frequently. Staff had to wear a lot of personal protective equipment to care for them, and they were hot and uncomfortable. At one point, we had an elderly COVID-19 patient in our hospital. They were in the intensive care unit for 77 days. I can mention it, because it's on the public record. I talked to an intensive care specialist about this patient, because if the situation was different and we were overwhelmed by COVID-19 then difficult decisions would have to be made. Could we keep going with this patient on a ventilator? 'This really raises an interesting ethical dilemma, because we know from this patient's experience that we can potentially keep people alive for significant periods of time in the intensive care unit. But, if we are resource-stretched, how do we keep doing that?' they said.

I often reflect on the life-and-death decisions that we make in this profession. I remember a surgical patient with a time-critical condition who we saw on a ward round when I was working in a particular specialty. We had been looking after the patient for weeks. He was young. That day, the consultant realised that there was nothing more we could do to help this patient. There were last-ditch efforts that could be tried, but the chances of success were extremely remote. In those few minutes, it was decided. We would not try anything else.

'I'm afraid this is it. There's nothing more we can do,' the consultant told the patient.

The patient was not expecting that. He had no idea that his time was limited. I'll never forget the look on his face.

It was a mixture of shock and confusion. His family sat around him, trying to absorb what just happened. We left the room. Several days later, he was gone.

That decision was made within minutes.

Another time, our consultant was convinced that an elderly patient had reached the end of the road. He decided that it was time for comfort care only. However, the family pleaded with him to continue treatment for another day or two. He had a long discussion with them about the futility of treatment and encouraged them to let their family member go. But the family persisted, and it was agreed we'd give it one more chance. And so, we did.

Two or three days later, the patient recovered. They left the hospital to spend more happy days at home.

There are often discussions about attempting treatments with remote chances of success. A good example is the resuscitative thoracotomy, or clamshell. This is a last-ditch effort for certain patients in cardiac arrest. The chest is cut open to try to resuscitate the heart. It's not an elegant procedure.

Some doctors are against it. Others say that even though the chances of success are so remote, you need to be able to look the family in the eye and say that you did everything you could. I probably sit in the latter camp, but there is probably no right answer here.

*

Apart from the medical risks to people with disabilities during COVID-19, there were social problems, too. Those with disabilities were having challenges with simple things like accessing groceries. Supermarkets had restrictions on who could attend from one household, making it difficult for people to go with a caregiver. Some people hoarded groceries, which made matters worse. The federal government drove the distribution of codes that allowed priority delivery of groceries to people with disabilities.

The general public began to stockpile basic medical supplies too. Some of these were essential supplies that someone like me needs for day-to-day life. It all became challenging to secure.

People who were dependent on caregivers attending them faced another set of unique risks. If one of those caregivers became infected with COVID-19 or even came under an order to isolate due to suspected contact with an infected person, the person with a disability could lose an entire team of caregivers who would be considered close contacts. The only safe place for them would be a hospital. If the person with the disability themselves was asked to isolate, the only practical place to do that would again be a hospital. Being in a hospital for any reason increases the risk of complications for disabled people, including infections from things like COVID-19 itself.

Some businesses were quick to fire people with disabilities first. Therefore, economic participation became even more challenging. Access to routine healthcare was limited. Elective surgeries and outpatient clinics were closed, delaying important healthcare.

There was a lot of anger about the various steps that were taken to control the pandemic. Undoubtedly, the situation was incredibly difficult for many people. To find strength, I thought back to the world wars. In those times, people were encouraged to consume less, so goods could be used for the war effort. People made things for the war effort. Young men and women sacrificed their youth, their health, and sometimes their lives for their country and justice. Millions of people across the world faced hardship. For years much of the world was literally and figuratively on fire.

If those generations were able to get through those times to get us where we are today, then I decided it wouldn't be hard for me to make sacrifices to ensure that my fellow humans remained safe – even if it was just one person. What if someone told me that if I stayed in lockdown for a month, I could save someone's grandma's life by stopping her from getting COVID-19? Would I make that sacrifice? The answer is easy. I hope that for most of us, putting things in this perspective makes the sacrifice a simple one.

I even came across some disability support workers who were willing to put their wellbeing at risk for the person who they cared for.

'What if your client gets COVID-19? Would you leave them, or continue to care for them?' I asked one.

'I wouldn't leave them. I'd keep going,' they said.

Even though I already knew it, this conversation cemented in me that people who do jobs like this are unsung heroes. To them, it's more than a job.

Fortunately, Australia and its neighbour New Zealand initially travelled through the start of the pandemic reasonably unscathed for a little while. There was no overwhelming number of COVID-19 cases. The hospitals remained unburdened from the disease. People with disabilities were protected by virtue of limited community spread.

This all quickly changed with later waves, like the Omicron variant. The politics of the pandemic damaged the integrity of our response. The states began to argue with the federal government. In the end, people with disabilities again suffered.

Other countries didn't fare well from the start. One example was Sri Lanka. They did extremely well at the very beginning, with next to no cases. Then, hotel quarantine failures occurred. That seemed to have been a weak spot for many countries. Eventually, COVID-19 began to run rampant across the nation. Sri Lanka had limited resources, so countries like Australia began to send supplies like hospital beds.

India became a disaster zone. They had to deal with hundreds of thousands of cases a day. Other countries, including some South American ones, faced similar issues. Political instability followed.

The best laid schemes of mice and men, right? In an instant nature can destroy the things that are at the core of our existence. It can change the way we function as a human race. It can topple nations. It can corrupt economies. It can take life.

The creation of vaccines for COVID-19 was probably one of the most significant achievements in human history. Previously, pandemics have wiped out vast swathes of our populations. Now, we have the ability to defend ourselves in a timely manner.

When the vaccine started to be rolled out, my hospital was one of the first in the country to access it. I was among the first groups to be vaccinated, being a healthcare worker with a medical condition. When I turned up to the vaccination clinic, one of the lead doctors was floating around.

'Do you think that I'm the first person with a spinal cord injury to be vaccinated in Australia?' I asked.

'You know, you most likely are. That's a very interesting proposition.'

From that jab onwards, I had less reason to be concerned about COVID-19.

While waiting in line for the jab, I was behind a police officer. The line kept moving forward. After about 15 minutes, we struck up a conversation.

The officer's name was Johnny Ngauamo. He was born in Tonga. When Johnny was four years old, his father had sustained a spinal cord injury. The injury sounded worse than mine. The family moved to New Zealand after it happened and Johnny's dad spent his days in a nursing home. However, Johnny and his mother were deeply involved in caring for him. Johnny had a good idea of what life is like for me.

Johnny wanted a better life for his family. He saw sport as a way out. On many days after school, Johnny hit a tennis ball against the wall. He then developed a passion for rugby union. Johnny made it in the sport, eventually playing for Tonga. Following a career in rugby league, he became a police officer. Johnny certainly made a better life for his family.

'Do you remember standing? Do you remember what it felt like?' he asked me.

'That's a really good question. No one has ever asked me that before,' I said.

'The reason I ask is because I've never seen my father walk. I just don't remember it.'

What you learn about a person is amazing, if you are open to it. Johnny had an incredible life. But he got me thinking as well. I don't remember what it feels like to walk. I do remember what it feels like to stand.

To be exact, I remember the last thing that I did standing. I hugged my mum. That is something I hope to be able to do again one day.

12

A RICH MAN COUNTING BLESSINGS

He is a wise man who does not grieve for the things
which he has not, but rejoices for those which he has.

Epictetus

MANY OF US have our hopes crushed because big dreams
are often said to be unrealistic. How many times have you
heard that? 'It's just never going to happen.'

In his book *The Diamond Cutter*, Michael Roach talks
about diamonds. A diamond is a dirty shapeless rock when it's
pulled out of the ground. There is no beauty to it. But when
cut perfectly, light travels perfectly through it. The diamond
sparkles. Reality is like that too. Every experience in life is like
a diamond pulled out of the ground. We can cut it into any
reality that we want. And if we are doing the cutting, why
should we accept someone else's version of what's realistic?

Will Smith said that '[b]eing realistic is the most

common path to mediocrity'. Being realistic isn't going to get us anywhere. And if someone says that it's unreasonable to be unrealistic, they are wrong too. George Bernard Shaw adds that a reasonable person adapts themself to the world. The unreasonable one persists in trying to adapt the world to themself. Therefore, all progress depends on the unreasonable ones.

And as Marianne Williamson once wrote, 'Our deepest fear is not that we are inadequate. Our deepest fear is that we are powerful beyond measure. It is our light, not our darkness, that most frightens us. We ask ourselves, Who am I to be brilliant, gorgeous, talented, fabulous? Actually, who are you not to be? You are a child of God. Your playing small doesn't serve the world.'

We need to be fearless. We need to dream big. We must be unrealistic. Unreasonable.

I was unrealistic about medical school. I was unreasonable about working as a doctor. Thankfully, it paid off. I'm unreasonable and unrealistic about curing paralysis too.

From the moment the accident happened, I had hope. I spent months, maybe years, trying to move my toes. I willed it in my head. I believed I could do it. I got some sensory function back. The first thing I felt was a toe. Then, I felt my booty. Tiny bits of sensation returned to parts of my body. None of it felt normal. As more time went on, I ran into every shaman, monk, charlatan and leprechaun that crossed my path.

People came to my place and prayed. Some danced around and carried out weird rituals. One fell asleep in a chair mid-ritual. I watched him snooze for a little while, then woke him up. Thank you for your hard work. Don't call me, I'll call you.

I can safely say that I've tried everything. I wanted to do anything I could to walk again.

I still see many people take this journey. Crowdfunding efforts raise money for the injured to go to the furthest corners of the earth with the hope of being cured. Stem cells in Panama. Activity therapy in the United States. Hyperbaric therapy in Melbourne. Ayurveda in India. Surgery in China. Millions of dollars for hope. While there are those exploiting vulnerable people, I still think that on balance it is better to let someone have hope. Hope got me through the hardest of times early in the injury.

In the never-ending hope for a cure, I've kept an eye on the science over the years. At the time of the accident, a large part of the focus on spinal cord injury revolved around stem cells. The idea was that stem cells would grow into nerves that reconnected the spinal cord. There wasn't much success. Some studies got to the point of growing new nerves from stem cells, but they weren't functional.

There once was a patient in Poland who regained function after getting a transplant of stem cells from their nose. These cells are thought to have potential to support spinal cord regrowth. I talked to a scientist about this one day and asked if this therapy could be quickly trialled further in Australia.

'No, it's too risky. If you take cells out of the nose, a person can lose up to 50 per cent of their sense of smell. This can make people depressed. And what if they don't smell a fire in time? How will they escape?' she said.

We got into an argument about the merits of such work, but she was adamant.

Think about it. People with spinal cord injuries are paralysed. *Paralysed.* They face so many physical and social challenges. Add to that depression, which is one of the biggest problems affecting people who experience spinal cord injury. The suicide risk is higher. And fire? Am I going to be able to run away from a fire if I smell it?

Ironically, most of the researchers in the scientific community aren't affected by the conditions they work on. They're disconnected from the lived experiences. I can tell you that if you haven't experienced depression, it's a very hard thing to fathom. Similarly, I have no idea what life is like for a person who is blind, a person who is deaf, or a person who is experiencing a stroke. So if I don't know, how can I ever develop meaningful, relevant research to help such conditions without engaging these very people?

With this sort of research, there's often no urgency for results, either. In the research world, scientists get paid a salary from money raised for research. This is fair because their expertise needs to be remunerated. But this system doesn't encourage quick outcomes. Scientists spend a great deal of time getting a grant, then spend more time applying for the next grant. The grants keep the money flowing in to pay salaries, but grants have a limited lifespan. Scientists also have other institutional targets to meet like publishing a certain number of papers annually. The more prestigious the journal, the higher the kudos.

The number of papers alone is sometimes judged as meaningful research output when it's not. In medicine, too, doctors are sometimes expected to publish papers to access specialty training programs. These programs have scoring systems for entry, where a paper might be worth a certain number of points. In some entry pathways, even the most meaningless paper will attract points. And there are many meaningless papers floating round.

For example, there was once a study conducted to see whether rats can discriminate between the Japanese and Dutch languages when they are played backwards. The rats couldn't tell the difference. What benefit this has for humanity when people are dying of all sorts of diseases, I don't know.

Similarly, the study outlined in the paper 'People's clothing behaviour according to external weather and indoor environment' found that people wear warm clothes when it gets cold outside. Ground-breaking. Another study exploring the side effects of sword swallowing found that the activity can cause injury to people. Call the Nobel Prize committee!

Search for pointless scientific studies on the internet sometime. You'll be surprised. It's entertaining, but the problem is, precious limited resources are being used for questions like these. We are spending billions of dollars on research. Resources need to be used more efficiently in the scientific world. We need results on things that matter.

As a general comment, whether in Australia or overseas, research projects can suffer from clashes of egos, and from people not wanting to collaborate, which in turn again impedes the efficient use of resources. Many researchers want to carve out the territory, build an empire, and be the first to do it. I had a phone call with one Australian scientist once. I wanted to talk to them about collaborating on a particular project. First, they denigrated me for being in medicine, which is apparently an age-old rivalry between academic researchers and clinical medicine. They then berated me for being so junior and attempting research. They had no interest in collaborating with me or anyone else. The last I heard, a multimillion-dollar project had come to a halt because this scientist's ego had caused a significant amount of friction with partners. Of course, the only people who really suffer from this infighting and delay are those in the spinal cord injury community experiencing paralysis.

With so many broken promises, delays and disconnects, the spinal cord injury community struggled with hope. It had also lost one of the giants that pushed research – Christopher Reeve. Fortunately, hope was around the corner.

In the early 2010s, a scientist named Grégoire Courtine performed an experiment on mice. The team induced spinal cord injuries in the mice so that they couldn't move their legs anymore. After a period of time, the mice were given a cocktail of drugs. In essence, these were similar drugs to antidepressants. Then, the mice got electrical stimulation and walking therapy. Eventually, the mice were able to use their legs again. When an autopsy was done on the mice, the researchers found that the injured spinal cord had grown new nerves. It had thickened out again by about 45 per cent. So, the team found that function could be restored. The spinal cord could be encouraged to regrow. Plus, all this could be done with minimally invasive interventions.

This was exciting. Still, how many animal studies do we see? How many of them make it to humans?

I emailed Grégoire. I received a generic automatic reply. The email said that he was getting much correspondence about the study. He couldn't reply to each message individually. However, Grégoire promised to keep working on moving the science forward.

A couple of years went by. Scientists in the United States decided to try this technique on humans. In addition to the electrical stimulation, they used a very old drug called buspirone, which is used to treat anxiety. Interestingly, the spinal cord researcher I met in the US, Professor Yang Teng (known as Ted), had done some of the earliest work with the drug. Buspirone acts on a specific neurotransmitter.

In addition to helping anxiety, the same neurotransmitter has been shown to affect motor function through the spinal cord.

Lo and behold, their study had the same effect as Grégoire Courtine's. People were able to move their limbs again after being paralysed for many years. A key scientist behind the work, Reggie Edgerton, said that this was the Model T Ford stage of the science. There was still much work to be done on improving it.

Around the same time, some scientists at America's Duke University took an entirely different approach. They started training people to walk in a virtual reality environment. A paralysed subject wore a virtual reality headset. Inside, they could see an avatar of themselves. The avatar was controlled by electroencephalograms – signals reading brainwaves. Essentially, a headset read the person's thoughts. When the person thought about walking, their avatar started to move around in the virtual reality environment. As they took a step, vibration devices delivered the step-like sensation to areas in the body where the patient still had sensation.

After training in virtual reality environments, the patients eventually graduated to assisted walking devices. In this way, completely paralysed patients regained some motor function.

These studies suggest that the spinal cord is able to rewire itself under the right conditions. We never believed that possible previously. As long ago as the 17th century BC, an Egyptian papyrus read: 'one who has a crushed vertebra in the back of his neck, and he is unaware of both his arms and legs, and is stuporous, this is a medical condition that cannot be healed'. Nothing changed in the thousands of years that followed. We have been able to keep paralysed people alive for longer since the mid-1900s, but there hasn't been a reproducible workable therapy for spinal cord injury recovery. Suddenly, there was hope.

Towards the end of medical school, I lived in an apartment building. Across the hall was a fellow medical student and down the hall was an Italian biomedical engineer. He was a researcher and went to the same university as me. I often wandered past his apartment and smelled the aromas of rich Italian food.

One day, we met in the lift. The guy was tall, with an Italian accent. His name was Claudio Pizzolato. Claudio and I became friends. We were around the same age and we had similar interests. When we spent time together, we talked about science. Naturally, our conversations gravitated towards spinal cord injury. I spoke to him about some of the advances that were happening in the field.

We started playing around with equipment. We even randomly found an electroencephalogram headset in someone's drawer at the university one day and the owner lent it to us to experiment with. We quickly realised that the science happening in the United States could be developed here in Australia, with our own unique twist. Our idea was to develop thought-controlled electrical stimulation and virtual reality rehabilitation paradigms combined with drug therapy. It's a mouthful, but the idea puts together all the science that has shown promise overseas. We wanted to use electrical stimulation to drive the limbs and maybe the spinal cord, driven by thought control using a headset that was readily available in the market. Someone would think about moving, then their limbs would be zapped into action. First, our plan was to train people to move their limbs in a virtual reality environment. Then, we would graduate them on to other things like exoskeletons – machines that help people walk. We planned to also use the drug buspirone. We called the idea BioSpine.

And so, in our own time, Claudio and I developed a proof of concept. We knew we could make it work. It was proper dirty citizen-led garage science. But we didn't have the resources to really take it forward.

Remember how I learned to say yes to everything? Well, that led to our next big break, through another sliding doors moment.

Greg, the friend who got married when I was in hospital and for whom I was a groomsman, was now the president of the Australian Lawyers Alliance. Greg asked me to do a talk for their annual conference, and I agreed.

The talk revolved around my life, my journey, and the

challenges that someone with a disability can experience. Towards the end of my speech, I highlighted the work Claudio and I were doing. I said that the dream to walk was coming closer; that therapies for paralysis were in sight.

There happened to be a man in the audience named Neil Singleton. Neil was the Motor Accident Insurance Commissioner, or MAIC. The MAIC invested in a range of programs to deal with the effects of motor accident trauma. The programs included cutting-edge research like stem cell therapy for spinal cord injury. Neil and I talked after my presentation. I sent MAIC a proposal outlining our work.

After that, MAIC asked us to make their staff a presentation at a room in the Princess Alexandra Hospital. It's where I was a patient after the accident. Claudio and I explained our work and our vision for the future. To build a foundation to one day carry out a human trial of BioSpine, we needed some resources. MAIC allowed us to lodge an application for a grant, which we did.

This road wasn't without tricky choices. As our project picked up steam, I got an offer to train in radiology at the Princess Alexandra Hospital. The hospital had a great radiology department who welcomed me. Many people apply for radiology. When I got my offer, something like six applicants in Queensland were chosen. It was competitive. It was like winning the lottery. The five-year training program would ensure a career that would provide security for Mum and me. But I would need to give up everything else to get through the training program – including the spinal cord injury research.

I thought long and hard. It was a choice between security and risk. Security was important. Mum and I had been through a lot. We experienced times where we had nothing, and I didn't want to be there again. Taking risk, however, could have a great payoff. I might be doing work that helps me walk again one day. It was a difficult decision.

In the end, I decided to take the risky road. I chose to kick on with the research, but also keep building the disability advocacy work which was gaining momentum. I discussed my choice with the Princess Alexandra Hospital's head radiologists. I was nervous about the meeting, expecting a difficult response. After all, they invested a lot of time planning to enable me in their department. My heart warmed when they supported the decision, knowing that it was the right thing for me. I learned that at the end of the day, good people will always support what's best for someone else.

Some time later, MAIC approved the grant. Our dream was going to come to life.

These days, I split my time between being a doctor in the emergency department, a researcher, disability advocate and lover of life.

How can I not love life?

In 2021, I became the Queensland Australian of the Year. It has been the biggest privilege of my life to date. I still can't believe that everything that has happened to me and everything I've done has culminated in this accolade. It's given me pause to think about a great many things. Firstly, I don't think that an Australian of the Year award is an award at all. Instead, it's a reminder of the journey that has been; a reminder to hold myself to a high standard. It's a reminder that I just need to keep going. Most importantly, it's a reminder that I need to keep giving.

The word 'Australian' has given me food for thought as well. I wasn't born an Australian, but I am a proud Australian today. What does it mean to be Australian, though? I love the Aussie philosophy of everyone deserving a 'fair go'. There's a lot in that phrase. It means that people have a go – they attempt things. They try. They persevere. And in my experience, they do. However, the idea has its roots in fairness. We support each other to do things. We value equity. We want to enable everyone to have a go at whatever they dream, disability or not.

For me, 2021 turned into an amazing year. I met inspiring people, went to incredible places, and did something like 200 engagements including talks and interviews. I even had the opportunity to be painted. One of the paintings, after being entered into the Archibald Prize, became a finalist in the Brisbane Portrait Prize then made its way to the National Museum of Australia. Never in my life would

I have imagined that someone would want to paint me, let alone put that painting in a museum.

It was a blast.

In among all this, someone asked me, 'Aren't you tired of always being on?'

'What do you mean?' I replied.

'I mean, you have to be this person talking about disability rights, medicine, or research all the time. Isn't that tiring?'

I was fascinated by this question, because it wasn't tiring. I wasn't putting anything on. It was just me. After some reflection, though, I realised that some of us may in fact 'put it on'. A politician once told me that he's a chameleon wherever he goes. He is rarely himself. I realised that it's that kind of disingenuity that makes people dislike politicians. We have to be ourselves. If we aren't truly ourselves in this world, it's a fast road to unhappiness.

We have to squeeze every drop out of life. We have to seize the day. *Carpe diem*.

You don't know what sliding doors moment is around the corner. You never know what butterfly effect you can set off. Amazing things can happen if you're open to it. But, you have to open yourself to the world for it to open itself to you.

It took me a long time to open myself to the world after the accident. I hid away, healed, then gathered the courage to step out. Luckily, I wasn't alone. I had people who took that journey with me. People who took a bet on me. People who fought for me and prodded me to keep going. It's important to celebrate the people who invest in us.

In 2020, I had the opportunity to give something to the National Museum of Australia. It was to be an object of significance to me. I gave them one of my scrub tops. It had 'Dr Dinesh Palipana' embroidered on one side of the chest. The scrub top symbolises me. Medicine is at my heart. Being a doctor is a part of my identity. The scrub top was then signed by people who took my journey with me, because we are forever shaped by the people who touch our lives. It was signed by the firemen who cut me out of the car. It was signed by the surgeon who operated on me. It was signed by the academics who helped me through medical school. Most importantly, it was signed by Mum.

Mum gave up so much to help me. She is the embodiment of love. She is the definition of patience, dedication, perseverance and strength. I still don't know how she's managed to stick by my side for so many years. I'm lucky to have her.

Today, I'm lucky to have another 'her' as well.

I was working one morning when I noticed a cute new doctor fiddling around with the printer. I wandered over to say hello.

'Is everything okay with that?' I asked.

'I'm just trying to figure out this printer,' the doctor replied in a Scottish accent.

I asked her a bit more about herself. Like many doctors, she moved here from the United Kingdom to work in sunny Australia. I like to say that she came here to hit on me.

We were friends for a while. I got to know her. She's beautiful on the outside, but amazing inside too. Her mind dances with mine. She's smart. There's a fire inside her. She challenges me, gives me cause to grow. Eventually, we got together. When two people come together, it's important that they help each other fly, enable each other to feel totally empowered, but at the same time feel safe enough to fall. That's been us.

What's more, she and Mum get along. When my mum was sick, I saw my girlfriend's gentle nature shine in the way she dealt with Mum. What's important to me was important to her as well.

I was talking to my friend Jeremy Howick once about how Mum and my girlfriend get along so well.

'That's a great sign,' he said. 'Have you ever seen a mama bear around her cubs? They never let anything bad get near the cubs. They go nuts. So, if your mum likes her, that's a great sign that she's a good person.'

She is a great person. And you know what I realised? I was right about not having a 'normal' relationship together. We've had an extraordinary relationship together. I'm lucky.

I'm lucky to have this life too. Every day, I am grateful. I'm grateful to live in this country. I'm grateful for my ability. I'm grateful for the promise of a bright future.

Even though I have a spinal cord injury, I have been able to work in the busiest emergency department in Australia. I was admitted as a lawyer. I have some firsts to my name. I've soared in the sky, cut through the oceans, and been on top of the most beautiful of mountains. I've done things that I never dreamed of.

I feel rich, and not because of any material possession. I feel rich because of the people around me. I feel rich for the incredible memories I have in the bank. I don't remember how many hours of sleep I got. I don't remember how much money I've earned. I remember the experiences, laughter and smiles. I hope that I've left my small piece of the earth better than I found it.

And today, I've written the first draft of a book in about three weeks. How can I say that I'm paralysed? No. Now, I'm stronger.

ACKNOWLEDGEMENTS

THANK YOU, JEREMY HOWICK. Jeremy persisted in encouraging me to write this book. The seeds that he planted ended up being the sprouts that Jamila Rizvi nurtured. Jamila took me, a first-time author, and introduced me to the world of publishing. Without these two people, this book would not have come to life. 'We rise by lifting others,' said Robert Ingersoll. After everything that they do to elevate people, Jamila and Jeremy must be flying past the moon by now.

Doctor-authors Atul Gawande and Eric Topol took the time to respond to my curious emails about their books while recovering from a spinal cord injury, even being in the busy positions that they are. They sent me signed copies of their books. I'm grateful for their inspiration. They've shaped my thinking about what it is to be a doctor.

Cate Blake, the publisher who took this humble author under her wing and helped me every step of the way to bring this book to the world. She taught me the process, nuances, and road to writing a book. Danielle Walker edited